BRAIN BASICS

BRAIN BASICS

BRAIN BASICS

AN INTEGRATED BIOLOGICAL APPROACH TO UNDERSTANDING AND ASSESSING HUMAN BEHAVIOR

Robert A. Williams, M.D.

Brain Basics is a book for anyone
interested in the biological approach
to human behavior and mental
illness

Edited by Ellen Antill

Production services and book design by Laura Lawrie, Mesa, Arizona.
Production management, illustrations, and book cover design by The Cricket
Contrast, Phoenix, Arizona.

For any additional information, contact:
Biological Psychiatry Institute
5133 N. Central, Suite 107
Phoenix, Arizona 85012
Phone: (602) 279-1026
Fax: (602) 279-0838

Contents

Contents

Dedication

Brain Basics is dedicated to . . . the University of New Mexico School of Medicine—thanks for the opportunity to study medicine . . . to my sister, Elizabeth; . . . and to my daughter, Victoria.

Acknowledgements

Praise is noteworthy for Ellen Antill, the editor of *Brain Basics*, for her excellent job. Thanks go to the staff at the Biological Psychiatry Institute, Janet Eshenbaugh and Bernie Baggett; to Sir William Osler, Jr., M.D., an admirable physician model; and to my patients.

Preface

In man's brain the impressions from outside are not merely registered; they produce concepts and ideas. They are the imprint of the external world upon the human brain. Therefore, it is not surprising that, after a long period of searching and erring, some of the concepts and ideas in human thinking should have come gradually closer to the fundamental laws of this world, that some of our thinking should reveal the true nature of atoms and the true movements of the stars. Nature, in the form of man, begins to recognize itself.

Victor Frederick Weisskopf
Knowledge and Wonder

It is no wonder that there is such widespread public bewilderment about psychiatric illness. Poor transfer of knowledge between scientific/research experts in psychiatry and the general population is a major contributing factor. When data about psychiatric illness *is* available, often it is unscientific or too technical for broad comprehension. Furthermore, the very concepts on which psychiatry is founded are an admixture of factual and mythic elements. Add the fact that there is no general model of psychiatry to unite competing paradigms into one intelligible perspective, and the environment is ripe for confusion.

Whereas public awareness of fundamental scientific facts is fairly good, appreciation of definite psychiatric principles has been lost in the "knowledge gap" between neuropsychiatry and the rest of the world. Even among healthcare professionals, widely disparate opinions exist with regard to cause of psychiatric illness and efficacy of treatments. My original objective in writing this book was to help patients understand behavior. Since then, it has evolved into an offering for the public at large, designed to bridge the knowledge gap and dispel widely held misconceptions about psychiatry.

The neuropsychiatric principles and definitions presented here, based on the general psychiatric model (the medical model), are beneficial for everyone's understanding of human behavior and illness. Furthermore, it is essential for all of us to know that *there is no perfect brain and that all of us will face one or more forms of brain failure at some point in our lives.*

It is my hope, for example, that the principles explained here will provide a common ground for both healthcare specialists and patients to bring about more rational and effective medical treatment of brain disorders. At the same time, attorneys can use the principles presented in *Brain Basics* to effect more equitable applications of the law to cases involving aspects of psychiatry. In the corporate world, *Brain Basics* principles can assist administrators with implementation of personnel policies that are more sensitive to the impact of mental health on work performance. In fact, *Brain Basics* can help individuals from all walks of life better understand the facts about diagnosis and treatment of brain disorders.

The first step in closing the knowledge gap is recognizing psychiatry's shift in focus from theories on maladaptive psychological processes to research on medical diseases. This approach, which began to gain momentum in the mid-1980s, emphasizes study and treatment of *brain* disorders as opposed to *mind* disorders.

Mental health usually is assessed, nonprofessionally, according to specific types of *behavior*; that is, external acts that reflect brain activity. Few people realize that behavior is an active biological entity, not simply a collection of attitudes and physical or verbal responses. It is an outward manifestation of the health of an internal organ—the brain.

Because of psychiatry's former emphasis on dysfunctional psychological processes, it is not surprising that there is such general misunderstanding about behavior and its biological determinants, including such conditions as depression, panic disorder and schizophrenia. The public perception of a psychiatrist as a bearded, bespectacled physician/therapist who probes the dreams and emotional trauma of his patient, as the latter lies on the infamous analyst's couch, is—at best—a limited view and reflective of a completely unscientific approach to psychiatric treatment.

Many psychiatrists still base patient care on psychological determinants of behavior, such as stress, lack of parental love, childhood trauma, and gender jealousy. Gradually, however, others are approaching diagnosis and therapy guided by the medical model, which considers the impact of biological *and* psychological determinants. In order to determine the presence of brain abnormalities, today's progressive psychiatrist takes into account not only factors noted in patients' psychological histories, but results of comprehensive physical examinations and scientific testing, as well.

Founded on basic laws of science and precise research methods, the medical model provides a rational approach to psychiatry and eliminates a great deal of "mystique" surrounding the specialty. At the Biological Psychiatry Institute, clinical application of the medical model has enabled us to more accurately "engineer" diagnosis and therapy, while revealing new aspects of specific disorders and changing the way they are treated.

Many psychiatric patients who receive care according to a psychological model are treated without benefit of systematic guidelines. The medical model, on the other hand, provides a precise way to monitor the presence or absence of active illness, a step-by-step method to determine whether behavior is illness-generated or personality-generated. Ultimately, when patients are taught to discern this difference, they can become empowered by greater understanding and are in a better position to take more responsibility for self-care.

The purpose of *Brain Basics* is to educate readers about the basics of psychiatry, with particular emphasis on principles of behavior. The five primary educational phases include:

1. definition of foundational terminology and explanation of normal brain function
2. definition of brain dysfunction, its mechanisms and methods of identification
3. description of biological psychiatric or neuropsychiatric diagnosis, based on the medical model
4. explanation of the open model or the integrated approach to psychiatry
5. presentation of guidelines for selecting a biological psychiatrist and description of neuropsychiatric principles used with the brain model of illness

It is my hope to close the psychiatric knowledge gap by arming readers from a range of backgrounds and professional experiences with an integrative approach to understanding human behavior that will help them recognize behavioral disorders and identify appropriate therapy. Those who acquire a heightened comprehension of the value of psychiatry based on the medical model may be in a position to make more timely, logical choices regarding behavioral healthcare and to retain the services of a reputable biological practitioner, if necessary.

(Author's note: Readers of this text who have no formal education in or experience with psychiatry may wish to begin with the clinical material contained in Chapter 4.)

Robert A. Williams, MD
Director, Biological Psychiatry Institute
Phoenix, Arizona
March, 1998

1
The Medical Model for Psychiatric Diagnosis

It takes as much time and trouble to pull down a falsehood as to build up a truth.

Peter Mere Latham
Collected Works

The purpose of Brain Basics is to counter social stigma's and cultural fads.
Robert A. Williams, M.D.

Psychiatry is the division of medicine that deals with the diagnosis and treatment of illnesses that affect the brain. The medical model, which is the scientific model that is applied to *all* fields of medicine, provides psychiatry with a rational approach to the diagnosis and treatment of brain disorders.

Unfortunately, the psychological model of psychiatry has dominated the field for much of the 20th century. Most American cultural perceptions of and attitudes toward behavior have developed in response to this nebulous and inexact approach to psychiatry. *Brain Basics* presents the groundwork for a new appreciation of human behavior, founded on three primary principles of the medical model:

1. *observation*—systematic and reproducible observation of physical phenomena (behavior)
2. *review/definition*—review of observational findings and development of operational definitions to facilitate general understanding
3. *diagnosis*—formulation of scientific diagnoses, based on relationship between disease physiology and cause of illness

(Author's note: Readers of this text who have no formal education in or experience with psychiatry may wish to begin with the clinical material contained in Chapter 4.)

The text will also attempt to define psychiatric concepts as clearly as possible, in terms of operative applications. Because specific psychiatric terms often are vague and poorly defined, many individuals approach psychiatry with an understandable sense of confusion. Even definitions found in the American Psychiatric Association's *Diagnostic Statistical Manual* (DSM) *III-R* are obscure. For example, "psychotic" is defined as "gross impairment in reality testing and the creation of a new reality."[1] Since "reality" is not definable, this description is not operational or usable. In fact, it may apply as well to "creativity" as it does to "psychotic." While creativity *has* been equated with psychosis (or madness), such an analogy is false. Creativity results from a heightened level of normal brain activity, but psychosis represents the presence of brain failure.

In order to establish a basic model of human behavior, elemental definitions are necessary. One of the most important terms that is used throughout the text—"behavior"—may be one of the least understood. Its definition, however, is simple. "Behavior" is anything that reflects brain activity. Overt behavior is activity that is observable without special equipment (such as an electroencephalograph). The terms "brain failure" or "psychotic" are used to describe behavior that clearly represents brain dysfunction. Brain failure is physiologically based and is treated with medical therapies. Maladaptive behavior that is *not* the result of brain dysfunction is described as "neurotic" behavior and is treated with psychological therapies.

The brain is the organ system of human behavior. When failure of the brain reaches a level that prevents normal activity, it is designated as "abnormal." The same is true for all physical organs. If a small amount of abnormal behavior is present that does not significantly affect normal activity, it is called a brain "aberration."

Abnormal organic behavior is characterized by the presence of particular clusters of signs and symptoms. For example, when the heart fails, physicians look for a cluster that may include changed heart and lung sounds, ankle swelling, and shortness of breath. When the brain fails, physicians look for clusters that vary, depending on the area of brain affected. Senility, caused by failure in general areas of the brain, can cause confusion and forgetfulness. Depression, brought about by failure of the limbic system, can result in depressed or irritable mood, sleep and appetite disturbance, slowed thinking, decreased concentration, suicidal thoughts, and decreased capacity to enjoy life. One of the essential tools used by biological psychiatrists to assess behavior is the phenomenologic Mental Status Examination (MSE), which will be detailed in Chapter 9 (see page 195).

In terms of extended application of the text, it is assumed that basic definitions of brain function and general concepts about brain disorders as generators of behavior will withstand the passage of time. On the other hand, references to specific pharmaceuticals are avoided because of the fluctuating popularity of various medications. Likewise, only broad classifications of brain disorders are described because of the rapid advancements now being made in genetic technology.

The Rise and Fall of Biological Psychiatry

Biologically based psychiatry arose as a clinical specialty in the mid-19th century,[2] but was heavily influenced by faddism and mysticism, much like all other branches of medicine. It was not until later in the century that Sir William Osler, Jr., M.D., set the stage for modern medicine by delineating the basic principles of the medical model. This scientific approach to diagnosis and treatment of illness emphasized unbiased analysis and openness to different points of view.

Osler's theories also underscored the significance of education and direct observation as a means of changing beliefs about illness. Many of today's teaching traditions are based on these precepts. Daily hospital rounds, for example, are designed to help medical students learn in an unprejudiced environment. Likewise, autopsy participants are taught to set aside all subjective judgments and correlate cause of illness with clinical findings, based on a post mortem examination.

Psychiatry applied the medical model until the early 20th century, when the psychologically based models of Sigmund Freud and other psychoanalysts captured the collective American imagination. These theories were founded on the assumption that human behavior is a result of social and environmental influences, not genetic predisposition and brain function. Although none were ever tested for validity, they were believed to be true. Physical determinants of behavior were disregarded in favor of more seductive psychological determinants. The medical model gradually fell into disuse and finally was dismissed because the "mind" was not considered to be a "testable" entity.

Psychological models dominated the field of psychiatry until the early 1980s. During their lengthy period of influence, they provided all meaningful direction within the specialty and deeply affected attitudes held by both psychiatric professionals and the public at large. They also had a major impact on America's social mores, economy, and its legal and educational systems.

The influence of psychological theories on social opinion is, in general, greatly underestimated. Many people, for instance, consider suicide involving a "self-inflicted" gunshot wound to be a "willful act." In truth, most completed suicides are reflections of the behavior of mental illness, not deliberate choices governed by an individual's personality. Just as misinformed is the view that anorexic weight loss symbolizes a "refusal to maintain body weight"[3] and that an anorexic *chooses* not to eat. In reality, the inability to maintain weight is reflective of behavior controlled by mental illness.

Psychological theories, much like the length of women's skirts, are guided by faddish trends that fall in and out of fashion. Nevertheless, they still have a strong effect on public response to various behavioral disorders. Gender jealousy (specifically, "penis envy") was named years ago as a motivation for dysfunctional behavior on the part of some girls and women. Currently, codependence, sexual abuse, and family-of-origin issues are in vogue as contributors to dysfunction for both men and women. Actually, there is no scientific reason to link psychiatric illness with any of these elements.

A brief analysis of the nation's economy reveals a strong connection between psychiatry based on psychological models and funds generated by many American businesses. In addition to healthcare-related enterprises, the publishing and broadcasting industries—with their profusion of health-based magazines, books, audio/videotapes, and television programs—profit greatly at the expense of public faith in fads and misconceptions.

One has only to review the transcript of any courtroom proceeding to perceive how completely psychological terminology has infiltrated the American system of jurisprudence. Liberal use of such terms as "willful negligence," "premeditation," "temporary insanity," "justifiable homicide," and their dramatic effect on the lives and deaths of plaintiffs and defendants reveal the tremendous power that psychological models wield in the legal arena.[4]

The testimony of psychologists, who have no formal medical training and are not licensed to perform physical examinations, is regarded in some courtrooms as equal to that of psychiatrists, who are degreed medical doctors. Incredibly, certain legal officials are sanctioning decreased standards that give nonmedical "doctors" authority to practice medicine, instead of requiring increased competence from psychiatrists. This position only lends credibility to psychologists' demands for hospital admitting and prescription writing privileges, two practices that could have devastating effects on the quality of healthcare in this country.

America's educational system has invested so comprehensively in psychosocial models of psychology that there is no widely available curriculum featuring scientific principles of behavior. Most of the training received by professionals for whom it is particularly essential to understand such tenets (i.e., attorneys, physicians, social workers, psychologists) portrays, at best, an incomplete picture of psychiatry. New concepts are routinely omitted, rendering courses and references obsolete. Thanks to a widening movement in support of the medical model in educational settings, led by the National Institute of Mental Health, psychiatry is undergoing a renaissance. Much of the information necessary to participate in this renaissance can be found in *Brain Basics*.

A Threat to the Status Quo

The position of strength from which psychological psychiatry has operated for more than 50 years makes the reemergence of biological psychiatry difficult. Even so, during the last 2 decades support for the medical model has been expanding, not only through the efforts of the National Institute of Mental Health, as mentioned earlier, but also through the actions of committed healthcare professionals. Increasingly, it is perceived as the only scientific, and therefore accurate, guide to treatment of psychiatric disorders.

The first version of the DSM, published in the 1960s, was written in response to an increasing number of inconsistencies cited in American psychiatric research and treatment. Some of the most notable of these included:

- absence of consistent diagnostic criteria for determining illness
- widely differing percentages of patients in various diagnostic categories
- previously condition-specific symptoms that came to be recognized as symptoms of many psychiatric conditions

Since it was first issued, DSM has been revised four times in order to remain up-to-date with current psychiatric findings. More than ever before, these findings reveal a fundamental failure of psychologically based psychiatry to systematically diagnose and treat brain disorders. Although there are instances when psychological therapies can be helpful for certain psychiatric patients, the practice of basing the entire field of psychiatry on such therapies is an invalid one.

The general sense that psychiatry has been moving in the wrong direction began approximately 30 years ago and has become sharply clarified in the last decade, particularly in light of the persistence of most psychiatric disorders. Some of this country's most common and disabling conditions (i.e., alcohol-induced organic mental disorders, cerebral vascular disease, seizure disorders, traumatic brain injury) are results of brain dysfunction.[5] Because their incidence has not been measurably reduced through psychologically based therapy, the movement is gathering momentum.

In addition, because of the social stigma that accompanies many psychiatric disorders, notable benefit can be derived by connecting them with specific biological causes.[6] For example, hallucinations, mood changes, impaired memory, and confusion are frequently misinterpreted by the public as "imaginary" psychological problems. Individuals diagnosed with such conditions often pay a high personal and professional price when they are unfairly labeled "lazy," "witchy," "forgetful" and worse. In fact, it is a common practice among psychologists to conclude that patients are "in denial" if symptoms do not improve.

During the past several years those who favor use of the medical model in psychiatry have begun to express their opinions more openly. Insurance companies are refusing to compensate patients and psychiatrists are being sued for ineffective treatment; print and broadcast media are disseminating scientifically based information; and a few psychiatric residency programs are even promoting the medical model. In spite of accumulating evidence favoring use of the medical model, however, traditional psychiatry clings to psychological models and stubbornly resists any change to the status quo.

There are several reasons for such widespread opposition to universal reapplication of the medical model within psychiatry.

Threat to economic stability of psychiatry "establishment"

The old psychologically based system has monopolized the healthcare marketplace for more than half a century, and an intricate network of specialists keeps it running smoothly. Psychological psychiatrists, social workers, psychologists, therapists, and administrators, as well as the legal system, interact to perpetuate a nonmedical approach to medical problems, involving in- and outpatient care.

Minimal public awareness

The current psychologically based system is strongly established and well staffed by professionals with impressive credentials and experience, many of whom profit from the mystique surrounding psychiatry. Individuals who tend to be intimidated by this combination of status and authority may be unable to ask questions about diagnoses and prescribed treatments. If there is no awareness of alternative approaches to psychiatric diagnosis, there is no need to challenge existing processes. Popular faddish theories play a powerful part, as well, in preventing public recognition of psychiatry's biological basis.

Educational and professional limitations

The medical educational system is founded on old psychological ideals, and tenured psychiatry professors have a vested interest in upholding these principles. As a result, psychiatric training emphasizes psychotherapy as the primary form of treatment, a nonmedical approach to patient care. Also, many that choose to become psychiatrists do so because they are uncomfortable with direct patient contact. There is a great deal of reluctance to adopt the medical model, which requires physical examination of patients and interpretation of biological testing.

Grass-Roots Effort and Research Can Bring Change

In spite of the heavy artillery amassed against use of the medical model in psychiatry, its proponents continue to grow in number. As biologically based information becomes more readily available to the American public and healthcare professionals, the present psychological focus of psychiatry will change.

Psychiatry patients who have been treated for any length of time with psychologically based therapies may be among those who are most receptive to a new emphasis in psychiatry. They, more than anyone, can identify with the frustration of undergoing long-term therapy with poor or nonexistent results. First, there are the claims of success, then extensive and costly psychotherapy. Finally, when no relief from symptoms is obtained, patients often hear such damning phrases as, "You don't want to get well," "You *need* your problem," or "Just give up your problems." Frustration can be minimized when patients and the public-at-large understand brain failure and can seek biologically based treatment, when it is indicated.

It is a well-documented social phenomenon that the process of modifying deeply entrenched belief systems is slow and characterized by resistance. This is especially true when large-scale economies, such as the massive framework supporting psychiatry, are involved.

Although a permanent transformation of psychiatry may take quite a while to facilitate, the restructuring process already has been active for more than 10 years. One key factor has been missing, however—a high level of public awareness about basic brain function. If *Brain Basics* accomplishes its goal, readers will gain an understanding of fundamental brain physiology and comprehension of the medical model as the most appropriate approach for treatment of brain dysfunction. When the public uses its clout to insist on use of the medical model, adding its considerable strength to existing imperatives for a new direction in psychiatry, then conservative medicine—practiced at the expense of opportunities provided by modern medicine—will no longer be tolerated.

American revolutionary leaders from George Washington to Ralph Nader have depended on grassroots efforts to overthrow unfair and deceptive forms of control. They appreciated the power of an informed public in effecting change. While psychological psychiatry is not a repressive political system, it *does* keep thousands of patients imprisoned by mental illness with prescriptions for unsuitable methods of treatment.

Various types of brain dysfunction, like other types of organic failure, are being studied continually. Recently, two disorders—schizophrenia and obsessive compulsive disorder (OCD)—that previously had been considered results of toilet training problems were officially acknowledged as biological disorders. This conclusion was based on genetic research and represents the shifting emphasis of psychiatry from psychological theories to the medical model.

Professional research and public action can restore the medical model to its position of prominence in psychiatry. *Brain Basics* is designed to help facilitate that objective by organizing diverse scientific data into a clear, accurate format that can be easily applied by individuals from all walks of life. Only when Americans have factual information will they be empowered to obtain the most timely, rational psychiatric care possible and secure true mental health.

References

1. *Diagnostic and statistical manual of mental disorders*. 3rd edition (revised). Washington, DC: The American Psychiatric Association; 1987:404.
2. Yodofsky SC, Hales RE. Introduction. In: Yodofsky SC, Hales RE, eds. *Neuropsychiatry*. Washington, DC: American Psychiatric Press, Inc.; 1992:xx.
3. *DSM-III-R*, 544.
4. It is not the purpose of *Brain Basics* to explore complex models of behavior that could explain criminal behavior.
5. Yodofsky, xxi.
6. Yodofsky, xxi.

2
Basic Brain Function

We are an intelligent species and the use of our intelligence quite properly gives us pleasure. In this respect the brain is like a muscle. When it is in use we feel very good. Understanding is joyous.

Carl Sagan
Broca's Brain

Evolution, the physical nature of existence and the human brain—each is a wonderment. The use of intelligence as a source of power ("muscle") to help others is joyous and a pleasure.

Robert A. Williams, M.D.

Before initiating detailed exploration of brain failure and how it can be mitigated by biologically based psychiatric diagnosis and treatment, a clear comprehension of brain structure and function is required. The following discussion primarily focuses on physical elements of the brain and how they shape human behavior. The influence of environmental factors on human behavior will be more fully examined in Chapter 5.

The Brain's Support System

In order to function properly—in "homeostasis"—the brain must be housed, protected, fed, and cleansed. These vital tasks are performed by various parts of the brain's support system.

The **skull** provides the brain's external housing and contains **cerebrospinal fluid (CSF)**, a solution produced by specialized cells within the brain. CSF circulates continuously throughout the different chambers of the brain and eventually is absorbed by the venous system. It can be clinically analyzed, via spinal tap, for evaluation of possible central nervous system (CNS) infections.

Three layers of **membrane** comprise the brain's internal protective covering. Lying directly on the brain's surface is a very thin covering called the **pia**. The second layer is the **arachnoid**, and the heavy outer membrane is the **dura**. Generally, names of these membranes are used to describe bleeding sites. For instance, bleeding that results from a head trauma (a hematoma) might be described as "subdural" because it initiates "under the dura." The rupture of a blood vessel (an aneurysm) might be described as a "subarachnoid hemorrhage."

The interface between blood vessels and the brain, the blood brain barrier (BBB), forms yet another protective shield for the brain. Two sets of **arteries**—the **vertebral basilar system** and **internal carotids**—supply the brain with nutrients (oxygen, glucose [sugar], vitamins, and essential amino acids) and cleansing properties found in blood.

The carotids enter from the front (anterior) of the brain while the vertebrals originate at the back (posterior). Branches from both arterial systems converge at the base of the brain to form the **Circle of Willis**. This is comprised of anterior and posterior portions of the internal carotids and their connections with the posterior branches of the basilar artery.

Internal Structure and Function

In order to prepare for later discussion about the capacities of various areas of the brain, an overview regarding the neuron—the brain's fundamental building block—first must be presented.

At initial glance, the brain's cellular makeup, consisting of billions of neurons, is deceptively simple. Actually, the diverse types of neurons, their large numbers and the multitude of neuronal connection patterns are responsible for the endless variety of activities controlled by the brain.[1]

A single neuron, which may present in many variations, is comprised of a cell body (soma), a series of dendrites, an axon, and an area of pre- and postsynaptic terminals. Cell bodies, which can be fairly large, form the gray matter of the brain. Axons are long, thin extensions of cell bodies and make up the white matter. Dendrites can appear in numerous patterns and branch out like antlers to form areas of pre- and postsynaptic receptors. Chemical signals are sent between neurons by way of the synapse, which is formed by the presynaptic terminal of one neuron and the postsynaptic area of another.

In the presynaptic area, if the electrical signal is sufficiently strong, a particular neurotransmitter is discharged. Neurotransmitters are modified amino acids, the major component of protein, and chemically facilitate the transmission of information between neurons. One theory about neurons is that each produces

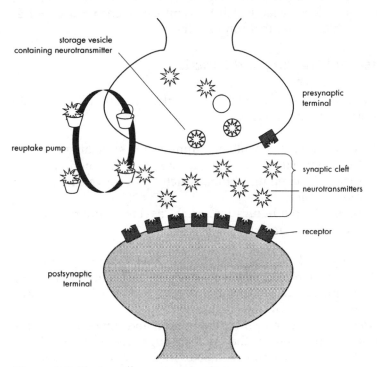

storage vesicle
containing neurotransmitter

presynaptic
terminal

reuptake pump

synaptic cleft

neurotransmitters

receptor

postsynaptic
terminal

Figure 2-1. Brain cell communication.

only one kind of neurotransmitter, but this is an obsolete view. In fact, neurons may produce a variety of neuro- transmitters. For example, one neuron (brain cell) may be characterized as serotonergic *and* cholinergic if it manufactures both serotonin and acetylcholine.

Because neurotransmitters are shaped somewhat like keys, it may enhance understanding to think of synaptic receptors as locks (Fig. 2-1). When the appropriate neurotransmitter is released, or "fits," into certain receptors, it can be compared to finding the right key for a lock. Once a sufficient number of receptors has been unlocked or activated, the cell body "fires off" an electrical current down its axon. This single electrical impulse, the basis for all brain activity, joins billions of other neuronal impulses to create human behavior.

The brain's top layer of tissue, the **cerebral cortex,** is comprised of neural cell bodies (gray matter) and axons (white matter) that conform to the humps (**gyri**) and valleys (**sulci**) of the outer brain.

Dispersed throughout the depths of the brain are clusters of neurons, called nuclei, which transmit electrochemical impulses via the white matter that connects them.

External Structure and Function

Utilizing highly organized networks of neurons, the brain coordinates four main tasks:

1. **Robotics**, such as walking, running, and stretching
2. **Cognition**, such as thought, awareness, and emotion
3. **External communication**, such as conversation and reproduction
4. **Internal communication**, such as life support and co-ordination of metabolic systems

Although physicians and researchers are beginning to understand more completely how sensory data enters the CNS and how instructions are communicated, relatively little is known about where and how data is analyzed.[2]

Examining the brain from the bottom and upward, we know that information enters the brain through the **spinal cord** and **cranial nerves**. The **brain stem** takes in sensory data and sends it on to higher brain centers. The **cerebellum** plays a major role in controlling fine motor movement. Above the midbrain lie the **diencephalon**, which serves as a relay station for incoming sensory data from the brain's periphery, and the **basal ganglia**, which is involved in coordination of fine motor movement and may play a part in behavioral response. The **thalamus**, adjacent to the diencephalon, is involved in sensory integration and movement, while the **hypothalamus** coordinates autonomic functions (heartbeat, breathing, etc.) and endocrine responses, such as those produced by the thyroid and adrenal glands. The four-lobed cerebral cortex, at the highest point in the brain, is comprised of the **frontal, parietal, temporal and occipital lobes**, which are divided by deep indentations, or **fissures** (Fig. 2-2).[3]

Neurons located in the four lobes of the brain control the following higher, more sophisticated cognitive functions of the brain:

Frontal lobe   *abstract thought
                                *awareness

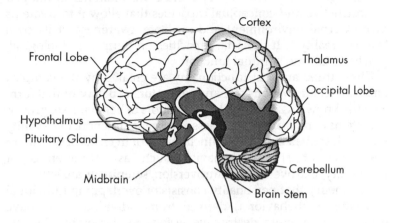

Figure 2-2. The brain.

	*motor skills
	*problem-solving
	*social functions
Parietal lobe	*gesturing
	*humor
	*ability to copy shapes
	*language
	*mathematics
	*vision
Temporal lobe	*musical appreciation
	*sense of rhythm
	*language
	*spirituality
	*hearing
Occipital lobe	*vision

The Brain's Interaction with Its Environment

Housed in the human skull, the brain is an isolated organ that has no direct contact with the outside world. It evolves continually as an extension of environmental influences and interacts with them in countless ways to impact personal and public life.

Throughout the evolutionary process, the brain has developed reconstructive and conceptual capacities that allow it to create its own external environment and facilitate awareness of its own "virtual reality." It reflects capacities in terms of biological, psychosocial, and spiritual function.

These three areas of functionality are created by the complex and parallel interactions of many **generators of behavior** that form a matrix known as **personality**. Generators of behavior are groups or systems of neurons that possess a common function. Personality may be described in terms of functionality or in terms of dominant generators of specific behavior, such as intuitiveness or practicality, extroversion or introversion, serenity or anxiety.

The theory that personality consists of overlapping individual generators of behavior is derived from individuals who have experienced discrete destructive lesions in the brain. Discrete lesions may result from strokes, small tumors, aneurysms, gunshot wounds, head trauma, etc. With certain discrete destructive lesions, one element from an individual's personality can be removed (i.e., the ability to add or subtract numbers [left parietal area] or the ability to express or appreciate humor [right parietal area]). Thus, it is surmised that personality is the matrix or composite of all the generators of the brain.

Brain failure is the inability of one or more of the brain's generators of behavior to operate within the personality matrix. In other words, the generator of behavior begins to create behavior that is *independent* of the personality structure. Generally, mild forms of brain failure occur when only one independent generator of behavior is affected and partially detached. In such cases, psychologically based (cognitive) therapy may be most useful in helping the brain regain control. As illness impacts other generators of behavior and overflows into new parts of the brain, biologically based treatment becomes more appropriate.

The main difference between psychiatry's current psychological focus and a biological emphasis is that the former relates illness to personality. Symptoms that arise independent of personality, as a result of failure of a generator of behavior, are the basis of psychiatry based on the medical model (psychopathology).

The three primary spheres of brain function that blend to create individual behavior also comprise the behavioral patterns of our society. When each sphere is stable and overlaps in a balanced fashion, psychiatry classifies behavior as "normal."

Biological sphere

When all areas of the brain are physically healthy and operating efficiently, biological balance is possible. Various types of disease and trauma can destroy stability in this area, sometimes with devastating effects.

Stroke is one of the most familiar causes of biological imbalance and commonly affects brain centers that control speech and muscle control. For many years it was assumed that depression following stroke was a psychologically based reaction to the physical insult. Now it is known that stroke, depending on its location and size, can produce *any* psychiatric syndrome. Therefore, poststroke depression—a biologically based phenomenon—is determined by the lesion's location, with injury to the left frontal lobe producing the greatest increase in depressed behavior. Contrast this with the absence of depression in automobile accident victims who manifest the same types of disability as stroke victims, but experience no head trauma.

Psychosocial sphere

Human beings are primarily social creatures who seek the companionship of others. Under balanced conditions the brain strives to preserve orderly social interaction, and guilt is one of the main mechanisms that helps maintain stability in response to socially accepted norms. Contemplation of antisocial acts (theft, murder, adultery, etc.) produces sufficiently strong fear and anxiety in the normally functioning brain to prevent actual expression. Threat of legal consequences, public shame and loss of status also exert powerful regulatory forces.

Excessive guilt and the absence of guilt can cause psychosocial imbalance. The former, which often is a byproduct of hyperreligiosity, may produce individualized conditions ranging from extreme nervousness to paranoid delusions. The inability to discern right from wrong, on the other hand, can have massive and devastating effects on society, in general. Sociopaths, individuals who are incapable of feeling guilt, do not embrace societal norms and often ignore accepted standards of behavior. Gang members who practice antisocial activities or political extremists who support illegal tactics fit the sociopathic model.

Spiritual sphere

Individuals may find spiritual balance and direction through formalized religion or may develop a sense of internal harmony and appreciation for life in a variety of other ways. Healthy spirituality is characterized by the capacity to live in the present and focus, for the most part, on positive life experiences. There is a well-developed acceptance of reality, an awareness of the value of people and a desire to seek rational truth.

The impact of balanced spirituality on behavior sometimes can be underestimated. Unfortunately, it frequently is assumed that when the biological and psychosocial spheres are stable, life is complete. Without spiritual balance, though, the emphasis that many people place on control can be overpowering. Individuals who cannot accept the irrationality of life with some degree of flexibility often try to manipulate the outcome of every situation and manage the actions of other people. They may encounter lifelong frustration and anxiety that can, over time, develop into psychiatric conditions.

The Key to Understanding Human Behavior

Although the brain never comes into direct contact with the outside world, it governs all existence and defines our awareness of reality. When the brain is healthy, it recognizes external information, processes it in the awareness center of the frontal lobe and translates it into internal perception . . . or the process may be reversed, from internal awareness to external action.

The world is represented in the brain because we have the capacity to perceive three-dimensional space and time. In this way, the brain functions as an extension of the environment. At the same time, the brain can exceed known reality and its own physical boundaries through insight and imagination.

The ability to remember, feel compassion, take risks, anticipate future requirements, ask questions and discover answers, create sophisticated technology never dreamed of before . . . this is the miracle of the brain, billions of neurons connecting with the world. The brain is the organ system of existence and the key to understanding human behavior.

References

1. Henn FA: The neurobiologic basis of psychiatric illness. In: Winokur G, Clayton P, eds. *The Medical Basis of Psychiatry*. Philadelphia: W B Saunders Company; 1986:463.
2. Henn, 461.
3. Henn, 462.

3
Human Behavior Defined

Mankind will possess incalculable advantages and extraordinary control over human behavior when the scientific investigator will be able to subject his fellow men to the same external analysis he would employ for any natural object, and when the human mind will contemplate itself not from within but from without.

Ivan Petrovich Pavlov
Scientific Study of So-Called Psychological Processes in the Higher Animals

Research is needed to better understand human behavior and illness.
Robert A. Williams, M.D.

The brain is the organ system of behavior.[1] Therefore, behavior, in the broad sense, is defined as anything that reflects brain activity.

Defining human behavior, in its "normal" state, is a vast undertaking. In fact, the many facets of human behavior and the uniqueness of each individual make it impossible to effectively define "normal." The purpose of this text is to give readers a simplified explanation of the biological approach to defining normal human behavior.

Accordingly, normal behavior will be interpreted here as the absence of abnormal behavior or the capacity of an individual to function within socially acceptable parameters in all areas of human life. For example, a low IQ that occurs in individuals without a definable illness does not necessarily signify brain failure. Without accompanying abnormal behavior, it may indicate only an expected value on a normal curve.

Human behavior is the result of many generators of the brain, which combine to form a matrix called personality. Generally, personality traits are evaluated according to the ways in which they affect human functioning. For example, the Minnesota Multi-Personality Inventory (MMPI) utilizes extensive and detailed questions to determine whether specific personality characteristics are normal or deviant.

When one or more generators of behavior pull away from the personality matrix and function "independent" of normal brain capacities, biologically based illness (abnormal behavior) occurs.

Independent Generators of Behavior

Let us consider the relationship between suicidal thoughts and independent generators of behavior. Suicidal thoughts may emanate as adaptable functions of normal brain processes. These functions may, in turn, relate to the capacity to cope with stress or avoid extreme pain.[2] During the period 72–73 AD, for example, hundreds of Jews committed suicide in Masada in order to avoid severe torture and enslavement by the Romans. In the present day we often hear of elderly individuals who choose to die with dignity rather than suffer slow and painful deaths. These two instances reflect rational thought or logical human reasoning as a natural aspect of personality.

On the other hand, individuals with major depression may have suicidal thoughts that are generated independent of the personality matrix. Suicidal thoughts in the context of major depression are irrational, are not under the control of affected individuals and, thus, are abnormal.[3]

Abnormal behavior is the result of brain failure, or the brain failing in its normal capacities. Independent generators may manifest in different forms of abnormal behavior, according to the type and/or degree of brain failure:

1. **Behavior that is outside the normal range.** Psychosis, which falls into this category, clearly represents brain dysfunction and is exemplified by an individual who experiences auditory hallucinations (hearing voices when no one is near).
2. **Behavior that is inappropriate for a given situation.** Rage and obsessive-compulsive behavior illustrate this specific scenario.
3. **Failure in a behavioral system.** This is represented by "clusters" of behavioral characteristics. Limbic system failure, for example, would cause major depression marked by fatigue, despair and apathy.
4. **Behavior marked by a cognitive deficit.** This is caused by dysfunction in a specific lobe of the brain.

Some individuals may display genetic predispositions for certain generators, such as introversion or extroversion, which strongly influence their personalities. In such cases, each generator of behavior is a dominant personality feature, not a separate generator of behavior. Psychosis, or brain dysfunction, occurs when a generator of behavior becomes independent of the personality matrix.

Generators of behavior also may be assigned to particular spheres of influence or the way in which particular generators of behavior function. In this regard, human behavior is categorized into four overlapping areas:

- Self
- Social
- Biological
- Spiritual

The brain, as an isolated organ system, produces *all* behavior, which ultimately can be translated into electrochemistry. Therefore, all behavior basically is biological.

When we view behavior, we categorize it in terms of human function. Most behavior is instinctive, preprogrammed or nonlearned, and it can be classified into that which does and does not involve awareness. When individuals function well in *all* behavioral areas, they are said to manifest "normal behavior."

Awareness behavior includes actions that influence the self, such as positive thought, self-esteem and confidence. Social behavior molds the way individuals influence and relate to one another, one-on-one or in group/cultural situations.

Behavior that is outside the realm of awareness includes autonomic nervous response, neuroendocrine behavior, and motor system behavior that is responsible for maintaining life support systems and robotics. Spiritual behavior (i.e., faith), which is viewed as being part of both awareness and nonawareness behavior, involves attitudes toward existence, creation, and oneness with the universe or a divine being.

Primary and Secondary Behaviors

Behavior may be classified according to the basic definition of behavior—"anything that reflects brain activity." The following classifications reflect different modalities of measurement for brain activity:

- Overt
- Electrical/Magnetic
- Metabolic
- Neuroendocrine

Overt behavior, which is described more completely later in this chapter, is the primary form of functional behavior. It can be observed without special equipment or testing. Generally, it is perceived externally (i.e., facial expressions, walking, tactile sensations, speech) or internally (i.e., perceptions, thoughts, emotions).

The three secondary behaviors of the brain, which are briefly described below, do not contribute directly to human functioning. Secondary behaviors cannot be evaluated through observation but must be quantified by special equipment.

Electrical behavior reflects electrical activity of the brain (brain waves), and is measured by an electroencephalogram (EEG). The most notable kind of electrical brain activity is sleep, which is essential for normal brain function. Magnetic behavior of the brain also can be measured by special equipment.

Sleep comprises the only set of normal behaviors that is defined electrically. All overt behavior that occurs during sleep, such as rapid eye movement (REM), is correlated by the primary determinant of sleep—the EEG. In contrast with overt behavior, EEG test findings are secondary. Even seizure disorders (sudden abnormal discharges of neurons) are defined by overt behaviors.

Five stages of sleep have been defined by EEG testing:

Stages 1 and 2	Light sleep
Stages 3 and 4	Deep, slow-wave sleep
REM Stage	Rapid eye movement (REM) sleep

Although the precise nature and process of sleep are not well understood, researchers have observed that a typical sleep architecture exists and that the REM stage (dream phase) increases as sleep progresses through the night. Also, it has been established that sleep behavior is related to awake behavior in the following ways:

- Sleep is necessary for functional awake behavior
- Events that are recorded in memory during awake periods may be recalled during the dream phase of sleep

- Sleep problems can cause awake behavior changes; for this reason, sleep studies can be helpful in diagnosing awake behavior problems

Metabolic behavior reflects the rate of brain cell metabolism. Metabolic patterns can be measured directly through diagnostic brain scanning called positron emission tomography (PET). Indirect measurement by evaluation of metabolites (breakdown products of the brain) also is possible, but this method has not yet proven successful because of contamination of peripheral nerve neurotransmitters.

Neuroendocrine behavior reflects the brain's hypothalamic pituitary activity, that is, activity of two specific structures of the brain. The pituitary gland is a small extension of the brain located on the brain's underside. The hypothalamus, situated above the pituitary, controls pituitary hormonal secretions. Certain mood disorders, which can produce abnormal neuroendocrine behavior, can be determined by measuring levels of specific hormones and neuropeptides (chemicals) in the blood.

The Expression of Overt Behavior

As stated earlier, overt behavior is observed behavior that is "overt" in the sense that it is observed without special equipment. Overt behavior can be perceived externally (i.e., behavior from another individual) or internally (i.e., behavior from the same individual) through awareness of one's own behavior. Within the brain, behavior is perceived by the awareness center in the frontal lobes.

Awareness is characterized by dimensionality that is based on:

- **Content**—that which an individual perceives
- **Place**—the origin of perception (internal vs. external)
- **Time**—the period during which perception occurs, relative to the past and future

Internally observed behavior is typified as "subjective." Externally observed behavior, which can be measured by standardized examinations, is typified as "objective."

Overt behavior is a complex set of overlapping behaviors that make human beings unique. The major avenues for expressing overt behavior include:

- **Language**—Human beings have the unusual capacity to speak, write, and read in a very sophisticated manner
- **Motor activity**—Human beings can move the various parts of their bodies in coordinated and task-specific ways
- **Perception**—Human beings possess exceptional ability to perceive the world, especially in terms of time and space; the five perceptual modalities are hearing, sight, touch, taste, and smell
- **Belief**—Although it is an unconscious process, human beings can crystallize perceptions or ideas in the form of beliefs. The exact nature of belief creation is unknown
- **Experience**—Human beings have an endless capacity to experience love, hate, guilt, fear, and a vast array of other feelings

A large part of total brain function is represented by these five aspects of human activity. They are set apart from other overt behaviors for examination because dysfunction in these specific areas signifies psychosis or disruption of normal human functioning.

During the 1800s, when the science of psychiatry was in its infancy, brain dysfunction or psychosis was described in terms of overt behavior of the brain. If an individual appeared balanced in each of the five main types of overt behavior, he or she was considered to be "normal" or nonpsychotic. Major disruptions in these areas were believed to signify the presence of brain failure. For example, the hallucinations and delusions that traditionally accompany schizophrenia (or unusual experiences described by some patients of "brain waves leaving their heads") were considered obvious indications of brain dysfunction. Psychosis was believed to be specific or unique to schizophrenia. No other physical conditions were thought to cause psychosis.

Today, psychiatrists realize that psychosis is nonspecific and can occur in almost every psychiatric disorder. Furthermore, it is recognized that the physiology of the brain is the major determinant of overt behavior, not past psychodynamics or psychoanalytic determinants.

Behavioral Form and Content

The external content of day-to-day living ("good" days and "bad" days) can influence overt behavior, and varying stress levels can cause reactivity to that content. Many people describe their level of reactivity in terms of mood (i.e., "I'm in a great mood today!"). In reality, mood is the underlying and dominant physiological state that exists independent of reactivity. The sense of light-headedness or oppression that an individual feels is an affect that is superimposed on the foundational mood state (i.e., mood is to affect as climate is to weather).

Obviously, culture is a major determinant of behavior; to a large extent, it determines the content of our lives. Social generators of behavior are uniquely designed for social function so that the brain creates social reactivity and society creates the social environment. An example of this is the sense of modesty. Society defines the parameters of modesty, but the actual sense of *being* modest is determined by the brain.

Emotional reactivity also can be socially guided. For instance, western cultures tend to emphasize hedonism. There is a dependence on environmental stimulation and reactivity. Eastern cultures, on the other hand, tend to minimize external reactivity and enhance the internal environment.

Overt behavior can be expressed in terms of *form* and *content*. In this respect, it is much like the spoken word. For example, the content of a verbal phrase—"I want to go home"—can have many forms, according to the manner in which it is conveyed (angrily, mournfully, exuberantly, etc.). Form and content are found in a work of art, as well, when the content of a painting includes lines and color, and the form includes motion or rhythm.

The causal relationship between form and content of overt behavior can be exhibited in countless variations. Depression, anxiety, suspicion, and jealousy are forms (or manifestations) of behavior while the object of these emotions comprises the content. When applied to language, the left side of the brain interprets literal content, while the right side handles the form of information. Because behavioral form usually relates to biological processes or physiology of the brain, it generally is treated by a biological psychiatrist. Behavioral content, which typically relates to psychological processes and past/present life events, is treated by a psychologist.

While form and content often *do* occur simultaneously, these two elements occasionally can lose their coincidental relationship and take on an independent existence based on the physiology of the brain (i.e., biological illness).

When the brain functions normally, all generators of behavior in the brain function within the personality matrix. When individuals attend to proper health maintenance, the cyclical needs of all generators of behavior are satisfied. These needs relate to: (a) appetite, (b) exercise, (c) sexuality, (d) sleep, (e) social inter-action, (f) spirituality, (g) nesting instinct, and (h) psychological welfare. As individuals attend more to the maintenance of these generators of behavior, internal stress on the brain is reduced and personal health is maximized.

When all generators of behavior function within the personality matrix, form and content are coincidental. Normally, behavioral form varies to a certain degree in relation to the content of our lives. When one or more generators of behavior in the brain separate from the personality matrix, form and content lose their coincidental relationship. The major determinant of behavior then is no longer the content of an individual's life but the changed physiology of the brain (i.e., chemical imbalance). The content of an individual's life, however, may convey an illusion that content is important, as the following example illustrates: A 42-year-old dentist reported, "I am depressed," (form) "because I cannot hear well" (content). After treatment, the dentist reported, "I am not depressed, but I still am feeling bad about not hearing well." The antidepressant prescribed for him was designed to treat the form of the behavior—depression. The content of the dentist's life was unchanged, but the relationship between form and content became appropriate or coincidental.

Successful biological psychiatric treatment is based on two primary factors:

1. recognition of a separate generator of behavior (form)
2. treatment of the form

These steps ultimately facilitate physiological reintegration of separate generators of behavior within the personality matrix.

The Impact of Independent Generators on Personality

In Chapter 2 the matrix of behavior, known as personality, was discussed briefly. There is no definition of a "normal" personality, but personality can be classified in terms of dominant generators of behavior, such as extroversion, insight, cynicism, or deviant types of behavior. If a particular generator of behavior within the personality is maladaptive and disrupts an individual's capacity to function, then he or she is described in the following terms:

- **Neurotic** (manifesting maladaptive behavior not caused by brain dysfunction)
- **Possessing a personality disorder cluster** or group of maladaptive personality traits that satisfy DSM-IV criteria for personality disorder
- **Antisocial**, as in cases of pedophilia and exhibitionism

Personality features are difficult to assess because a single personality trait may be like a double-edged sword—adaptive in one environment and maladaptive in another. For instance, an obsessive perfectionistic individual may function very well professionally as a computer programmer but may find extreme challenge in interpersonal relationships.

Appendices A, B, and C provide examples of several different types of illness behavior and how they specifically affected career development both positively and negatively.[4]

When a generator of behavior creates activity that is independent of the personality matrix and affects normal functioning, "abnormal" behavior exists. The Williams Brain Model shows the relationships of personality behavior, content of life, illness behavior, and awareness (Figs. 3-1a, 3-1b, and 3-1c). The brain is complex, however, and occasionally can harmlessly "misfire" like a car engine. An independent generator can produce nondisruptive behavior triggered, for example, by a "small voice" inside the head. Generally, activity of this type—called "aberrant behavior"—is of no consequence. Most of us have had multiple experiences with responding to a voice we presumed was "real," only to discover no one else was present.

Therefore, an independent generator of behavior can reflect excessively low or high levels of activity. Deep within the brain are located groups of neurons called basal ganglia. The basal ganglia are part of a widespread matrix of behavior that facilitates human robotics (smooth, coordinated, functional movement). Insufficient production of dopamine (a neurotransmitter) in the basal ganglia results in Parkinson's disease, which is characterized by a motor behavioral cluster—slow movement, tremors, muscle rigidity, and gait difficulties. The net effect of this type of motor behavior, produced independently of the normal motor matrix, is too little movement.

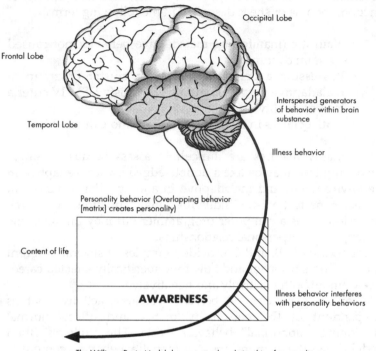

Occipital Lobe

Frontal Lobe

Interspersed generators
of behavior within brain
substance

Temporal Lobe

Illness behavior

Personality behavior (Overlapping behavior
[matrix] creates personality)

Content of life

AWARENESS

Illness behavior interferes
with personality behaviors

The Williams Brain Model demonstrates the relationship of personality
behavior, content of life, illness behavior and awareness.

Figure 3-1a. The Williams Brain Model.

The same system is used to classify neurological disorders (marked by an awareness of illness) and biological psychiatric disorders (marked by generators that create too much or too little of a particular type of behavior). Interestingly, movement disorders are divided into categories, based on awareness. The nonfrontal lobe awareness groups of movement disorders are subdivided into those manifesting excessive movement (hyperkinetic), such as Huntington's chorea, and those manifesting inadequate movement (hypokinetic), such as Parkinson's disease. As is the case in neuropsychiatric disorders, movement disorders are diagnosed by observing overt behavior or motor behavioral clusters (i.e., defining brain failure within the motor system).[5]

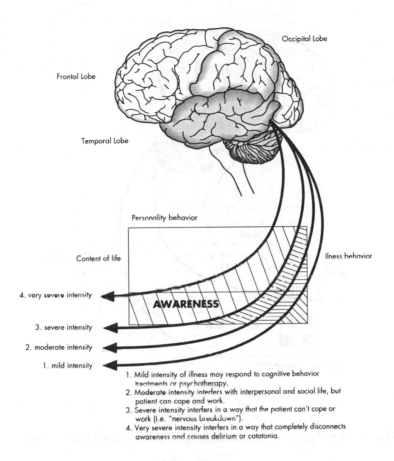

Figure 3-1b. Intensity of illness and the Williams Brain Model.

As is true in any disorders of the brain, when the brain fails, it produces excessive or insufficient behavior. Illness occurs when generators of behavior become independent of the normal physiological matrix. Disorders of the brain reflect either too little activity, as seen in attention deficit disorder, or too much activity, as seen in mania.

Brain failure is secondary to the presence of sick neurons or brain cells, just as heart failure is secondary to sick heart cells. Brain failure may be viewed as a "chemical imbalance" within neurons that alters the amount of behavior within a generator of behavior. As a generator of behavior becomes independent, it loses its

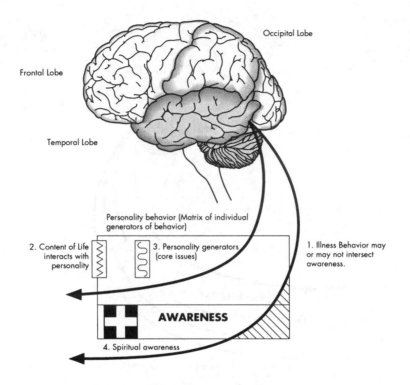

Figure 3-1c. Open diagnostic model and the Williams Brain Model.

normal ability to interact with other parts of the brain. Illness results when an independent generator of behavior interferes with normal human functioning.

Examples of too much or too little brain phenomenology can be cited in *all* brain disorders. Formalized medicine, however, places an unrealistic division between neurological and psychiatric problems. There is no difference, as the following paragraphs illustrate.

In terms of neurological disorders, Parkinson's disease results when too little dopamine is present in the basal ganglia; attempts to correct the disease by increasing dopamine levels may increase dopamine in other parts of the brain and cause hallucinations. In schizophrenia, which may be characterized by hallucinations, too much dopamine is present in certain parts of the brain. When attempts are made with antipsychotics to block dopamine production in one part of the brain, dopamine production in the basal ganglia may be inhibited, thus causing Parkinson's syndrome.

In terms of psychiatric disorders, there are many examples of diseases that typify the too-much/too-little generator concept. Posttraumatic disorder, for example, is the result of too much memory. Alzheimer's disease is the result of too little memory.

Finally, the more advanced a disease process becomes, the greater number of independent generators are involved. In the initial stages of Alzheimer's disease, for example, generators of behavior in the hippocampus (which governs memory) and parietal lobes (which govern sense of location) typically are the most sensitive. As brain failure progresses, some patients also experience depression (involving generators in the limbic system) or psychosis (affecting generators in the temporal lobes).

Awareness of Abnormal Behavior

Cosmologists and other researchers view awareness as one of the keys to understanding our universe. The human brain has evolved with the capacity to reconstruct the physical world, to be "aware" of time, space, and matter. As such, the brain is a reflection of the outside world and reveals essential insights into existence.

Awareness, the main components of which occur in the brain's frontal lobes, is a sustained thought that produces simultaneous associations based on the following process:

- active perception
- assignment of emotional coloring
- autonomic reactivity
- mood reactivity
- triggered memories
- sense of time

As one element of normal neurological functioning, awareness usually reflects the status of overall brain function. For example, when there is awareness of hunger, eating is the normal cognitive response. When individuals are overwhelmed with sadness or joy, they may respond emotionally with tears.

When behavior becomes independent of the personality matrix, abnormal behavior may not filter through the awareness center. Patients may not have the capacity to recognize their abnormal behavior. In neuropsychiatry, we characterize these patients as lacking insight into their illness; in psychology patients are said to be "in denial." It is inappropriate, however, to equate lack of insight (a physical process) with denial (a theoretical psychological process).

In fact, "denial" is a defense mechanism, an "automatic psychological process that protects individuals from anxiety and from awareness of internal or external stressors or dangers" (DSM-IV). As a physical process, denial can manifest as a result of two processes:

1. **circumvention of awareness**—In this case, behavior circumvents frontal lobe awareness and patients have no capacity to see their illness. This frequently is true for individuals who have addictive or manic disorders. In order to treat patients who practice this type of denial, it is most effective to focus on the consequences of their behavior. Over time the development of trust between patient and psychiatrist can motivate the patient to formulate an illusion-free belief process.

2. **active cognitive process**—Here, behavior is based on omission of undesirable thoughts from the awareness center. This typically applies to cases of mild depression, mild anxiety, mild migraine headaches, and other disorders. The active cognitive process used to remove unwanted thoughts or sensations can take the form of distraction (focusing on more enjoyable issues), meditation, positive affirmation, and prayer. Treatment is based on helping patients become more sensitive to the perceptions within the awareness center.

Patients who experience right-sided strokes have a lack of awareness in that they commonly fail to recognize their left-sided paralysis, a condition called anosognosia.[6] If there is no awareness that the left arm is weak, then there can be no purposeful intention to move it or motivation for rehabilitation.

Likewise, if there is no awareness of psychiatric dysfunction—as is true for patients with mania, addiction, and schizophrenia—there may be no motivation to seek assistance. Patients who have other types of illnesses, such as Alzheimer's disease, have varying capacities of insight into their disorders. I have found one of the most frustrating aspects of psychiatry to be the lack of motivation stemming from many patients' inability to "see" their illness.

The brain is the organ system of existence. "Existence" will be simply defined here as the interaction of mass, energy and time particles. Awareness is sustained thought that is produced in response to information received in the frontal lobe awareness center, the part of the brain that creates a sense of "existence." Disorders of awareness can play a role in illness in many ways.

Frequently, awareness or lack of awareness is mentioned as an aspect of mental illness. In movement disorders, for example, awareness is named specifically in the definition for Tourette's disorder, whereas lack of awareness is named in the definition for Parkinson's disease.

In psychiatry, a delusion is defined as a fixed false belief implying that an individual has no insight or awareness that the belief is false. Patients who have addiction disorders lack the capacity to see the addictive generator, often in spite of grave consequences. Patients with manic disorders may lack the capacity to see the absurdity of their outward behavior.

Hypochondriasis is another form of brain failure that can be notably frustrating, especially for general practitioners and internists. This disorder is typified by obsessive thoughts involving fears of having a serious illness. Resulting anxiety is based on perceptual difficulties in interpreting physical signs and symptoms, but hypochondriacs cannot recognize excessive fear as being a misinterpretation by the brain. In spite of reassurance by physicians, patients continually seek medical attention.

Awareness also can be characterized by behavior that relates to body or brain and reconstructions that relate to physical realities outside the body and brain. These are phenomena that are not yet fully understood by medical scientists. An example of this can be seen in Beethoven who, during his later years, was completely deaf. Reportedly, the composer could not hear his finished masterpieces but he could internally "hear" them perfectly well. Beethoven's creative genius included a marvelous awareness of dynamics, rhythm, and harmonics that allowed him to internally construct magnificent musical works.

Because the brain can fail in its usual capacities, brain failure patterns are predictable. *All* brain failure manifests itself according to one of three basic patterns:

1. Behavioral clusters
2. Presence of traditional psychosis
3. Specific lobe dysfunction

These patterns will be discussed later in more detail.

Determination of Awareness

Most individuals who are unable to recognize their own symptoms of mental illness are incapable of consenting to treatment. Because of this, often it can be difficult to determine an individual's awareness level and accompanying capacity to make decisions.[7]

Awareness is, in fact, a big "bugaboo" in psychiatry. Patients often manifest lack of awareness marked by one or more of the following characteristics:

1. inability to make medical or financial decisions
2. involvement in activities that are dangerous to themselves
3. involvement in activities that are dangerous to others
4. inability to care for basic needs of food, shelter, hygiene, or safety

If patients voluntarily submit themselves to a process of rational care, there is no treatment problem. If patients who exhibit one or more of the above traits cannot voluntarily submit to treatment because of mental illness, then legal measures can be instituted.

The next section provides guidelines for lay readers to measure awareness and competence in individuals whose behavior indicates possible mental illness.[8] These standards furnish a reasonable foundation for lay evaluation, but a professional psychiatrist is the only one qualified to establish a formal diagnosis after thorough examination of specific types of behavior.

Multiple Generators of Behavior That Are Necessary for Normal Function

1. Appreciation of the nature of the situation
Awareness is affected by space, time, events, and results when there is a sustained capacity to be cognizant of activities inside or outside the brain or body. A competent individual should be aware of:

- The presence of illness
- The need for treatment
- The consequences, if no treatments are received

- The physician's role in the treatment process

2. *Understanding of the issues related to treatment*

Acquisition of information and comprehension requires both long- and short-term memory. A competent individual should be aware of:

- Treatment benefits
- Treatment risks
- Treatment options

3. *Ability to rationally manipulate information and make choices based on practical reasoning*

Elements that might interfere with an individual's capacity to think and reason could include independent generators of behavior, such as depression or severe anxiety. The presence of these generators can nullify the following factors:

- Concern for personal well-being
- Desire to recover from illness
- Hope regarding improvement or recovery
- Absence of delusions regarding treatment decisions

4. *Ability to express a clear choice, either favoring or opposing treatment*

When an individual has awareness and understanding of the facts regarding treatment, and it has been determined that no independent generators are present, then decision-making ability can be evaluated. A competent person should be able to:

- Formulate and express a firm choice
- Prefer making his or her own decision
- Designate an appropriate surrogate, if necessary

Although competency is a complex function of the brain that can vary widely from hour to hour and day to day, all types of brain failure can be evaluated according to the preceding model. Whether the individual is anorexic, depressed, paranoid, or in the midst of a panic attack, the same questions can be asked:

1. Is the individual aware of activities going on nearby?
2. Can the individual factually recall past events?

3. Are there any independent generators of behavior interfering with judgment?
4. Is the individual able to make choices?
5. Are neurological functions interrupted by psychosis or brain dysfunction?

Answers to these questions allow an opinion to be formed by one individual about the competency of another. Competency determination is not an exact or scientific method, but it is an important reference point in the evaluation of behavior. An individual is medically competent if the neurological functions for being medically competent are present and brain dysfunction that might interfere with those functions is absent. Medical incompetence exists when brain dysfunction is shown to interfere with the neurological capacities required for medical competence.[9]

The Role of Instinct

Because behavior in the brain is preprogrammed or instinctive, brain failure primarily reflects changes in instinctive behavioral patterns. The brain provides the instinctive form of behavior and society provides the content, in terms of values and traditions.

For instance, mating instincts give individuals the desire to be attractive to members of the opposite sex, but society defines the standards (content) of physical attractiveness. Many individuals for whom social guidelines are major stress-producers have susceptible generators that produce bulimia, anorexia, or other social phobias. Thus, it is theorized that certain social stressors (i.e., financial problems, physical unattractiveness, lack of popularity with others, etc.) decrease the threshold for development of specific illnesses. These disorders include acute stress reaction, demoralization syndrome, posttraumatic stress disorder, psychosomatic illness, acute brain effects (i.e., insomnia), and aggravation of an underlying psychiatric disorder.

Specific generators of instinct and the type(s) of behavior on which they have an impact include:

Generator of Instinct	Type of Behavior
Appetite	Biological
Grooming	Interpersonal/Social
Guilt	Social
Language	Social

Modesty	Social
Motor capacity	Social/Biological
Sex drive	Biological
Sleep	Biological
Social needs (companionship)	Social
Territoriality (sense of ownership)	Interpersonal

The grooming instinct can produce several varieties of disorders. Tricotillomania occurs when an individual becomes obsessed with twisting and/or pulling hair. A body dysmorphic disorder can result in an obsession with minor body defects and compulsive mirror checking. Individuals with an olfactory disorder believe that they are emitting unpleasant body odors. A multimillion dollar cosmetic and perfume industry has developed around the instinctive need to look and smell good, a phenomenon that is perceived as normal in our appearance-conscious culture.

The bonding instinct helps individuals share common interests and values, to feel commitment toward one another. When bonding between two people is interrupted, as in the case of divorce, a string of behavioral disorders may result. Territoriality is invaded, setting the stage for anger and jealousy. Insecurity sets in when financial stability is threatened. Disruption of social and sexual rhythms can cause severe stress and depression. Finally, grief over lost emotional intimacy may persist for an extended period of time. Thus, emotional instability can have strong biological determinants, even though the process appears psychological or social.

It commonly is heard that certain instinctive behaviors, such as sexual activity or eating, are addictive. Instinctive behavior, however, is *not* addictive. The instinctive desire for sex or food is normal and originates from a natural generator of behavior. Addictive behavior, on the other hand, occurs when part of the brain is challenged by a particular substance, and an unnatural independent generator of behavior emerges.

The unnatural independent generator creates an abnormal desire for a particular substance, a desire that never would have occurred without repeated introductions of the substance to the brain. Eating and sexual behaviors—instinctive, natural generators of behavior—can take many maladaptive forms that are highly disruptive to normal functioning. For example, both overeating and sexual promiscuity often are used as stress relievers. Because eating and sexual disorders generally manifest as undesirable compulsive behaviors, however, they are viewed somewhat as addictive disorders. In fact, these two types of disorders can be formally addressed in 12-step programs similar to those used by Alcoholics Anonymous (see Chapter 7).

Evaluating Behavior with the Mental Status Exam

Establishing the *major* determinant of behavior—biological, psychosocial, or spiritual—is one of the most important steps in making a diagnosis and planning appropriate treatment. This process can be accomplished by first ruling out biological influences, then evaluating psychosocial and spiritual determinants.

For example, when I counsel a married couple with regard to an interpersonal problem, I begin by evaluating each individual for biological illness. If the behavior of one or both is marked by irrational or independent generators of behavior that interfere with their relationship, I initially treat the biological illness. Marital counseling parallels the biological treatment.

In the case of a lonely and socially isolated patient, I begin investigating such biological processes as depression, panic attack syndrome, and social phobia. Counseling may supplement biological treatment. Elimination of biological processes involves systematic observation of overt behaviors and use of the Mental Status Examination (MSE), first mentioned in Chapter 1. The MSE is designed primarily to provide a basis for assessing current behavior. Behavior can be evaluated in terms of psychosis (i.e., overt behavior that clearly represents brain dysfunction) or behavior that may be normal when viewed as an independent activity but is seen as inappropriate in a social context. The mechanisms that stimulate inappropriate behavior define brain function.

For example, if an employee makes a costly error that strongly affects a company's economic stability, it is appropriate for the boss to be angry. If the boss overreacts to relatively small mistakes, however, such as mishandled phone calls or minor typographical errors, then anger probably is inappropriate. If an individual appears nude on the street, such behavior is deemed inappropriate, but the same behavior enacted in a bedroom or nudist camp is completely acceptable.

The MSE utilized in my clinic is based on evaluation of three primary functions:

1. **Observed behavior** (reveals the presence of behavioral clusters). Analysis during the first phase seeks specific signs of brain failure, which usually are found in behavioral clusters. The cluster often found with depression, for example, might include hopelessness, fatigue, inability to concentrate and memory loss. Findings are based on (a) appearance, (b) mood and affect, and (c) motor level.
2. **Queried behavior** (reveals the presence of traditional psychosis). Analysis during the second phase seeks specific signs of psychosis revealed through direct questioning. Findings are based on (a) perceptual disturbance, (b) language disturbance, (c) belief disturbance, and (d) experiential disturbance.
3. **Cognitive function** (reveals the presence of specific lobe dysfunction). Analysis during the third phase primarily is derived through testing and reveals (a) alertness and orientation, (b) memory, and (c) language capacity.

Occasionally, evaluation of a fourth phase ("special considerations") may be necessary. Involving analysis of legal requirements and physician responsibility to potential victims, this process item encompasses instances of suicide, homicide, severe disability, and patient threat to self and/or others.

The human brain does not reflect abnormalities on a continuous basis. Some brain failure is cyclical (depression), some is situational (anorexic behavior), some occurs randomly (severe insecurity), and some occurs during sleep (fear and anxiety). For this reason, the MSE is just one method of evaluating behavior. Beyond its limitations, direct observation of behavioral clusters, psychotic behavior, and specific lobe dysfunction is employed. A complete discussion about the MSE is presented in Chapter 9.

Summary

Behavior is anything that reflects brain activity. Electrical, metabolic, and neuroendocrine behavior can be measured in order to learn more about brain function, but overt behavior reveals primary behavioral patterns. Ultimately, overt behavior—as it relates to human functioning—defines normal human behavior. Absence of explicit brain dysfunction defines normal physiological or biological behavior. Abnormal behavior in the presence of normal physiological behavior defines maladaptive or neurotic behavior, as well as personality disorders.

Analysis of language, motor activity, perception, belief, and experience traditionally has defined psychosis. In fact, in the past it was believed that certain psychoses ("first ranked") defined schizophrenia. Now it is known that psychosis is nonspecific and simply signifies behavior that represents brain dysfunction.

Behavior is divided into form and content. Relative to neuropsychiatric disorders, physiology of the brain—not the content of an individual's life—is the major determinant of form.

Independent generators of behavior are defined in terms of behavioral clusters, traditional psychosis, or specific lobe dysfunction. Lack of awareness capacity also plays a role in mental and neurological illness. Awareness and competence can be measured in terms of an individual's appreciation of the nature of the situation, understanding of issues related to treatment, ability to manipulate information, and the capacity to express clear choices with regard to treatment.

Social expectations have a particularly significant impact on behavioral patterns that are motivated by instinct. Such instincts as appetite, grooming, sleep, and sex drive can be expressed through abnormal behavior, especially if social norms governing these areas are unrealistic or stressful.

The MSE is a direct observation of brain function, or a formalized measurement of overt behavior. The MSE defines brain dysfunction in one of three types of phenomenology: (a) behavioral clusters, (b) traditional psychosis, and (c) specific lobe dysfunction.

The biological psychiatrist primarily is concerned with defining abnormal behavior through an individual's history and through neurological and psychiatric mental status examinations. Biological psychiatrists also focus on maladaptive or neurotic behavioral determinants that contribute to stress, including health maintenance issues (i.e., sleep, eating, and exercise habits). The medical model, which is practiced by biological psychiatrists, is an open-ended, scientific, and rational approach to understanding normal human behavior.

References

1. Understanding of the brain as an organ system of behavior may be enhanced by comparing its composition, from the most basic element to the most complex, to composition of the entire human body:

Composition of the Brain	Composition of the Body
Neurons	Cells of the body
Ganglia (groups of neurons)	Tissues
Generators of behavior (systems of neurons)	Organs
Behavior	Systemic function of organs

2. Biologically determined suicidal thoughts, which counter the instinct to live, may lead to psychological processes that view suicide as a rational process. Informal social support systems that discourage suicidal thoughts include family and friends. Formal support systems, such as hospitals and suicide prevention centers are important for two primary reasons: (a) they help delay suicide attempts so that effective therapy can be instituted—although statistics reveal that suicide prevention center programs appear to be rather ineffective, this shortcoming is related more to the lack of meaningful therapy and not to any deficiency in the centers themselves, and (b) they may prevent epidemics of suicide; certain individuals who are vulnerable to the influence of the current suicide rate can be dissuaded from mimicking this behavior.

3. Following is the sequence of treatment for suicidal behavior: (a) Identify major determinants of suicidal behavior (i.e., depression or psychosis) and initiate treatment; (b) Treat acute symptoms, including insomnia, anxiety and agitation; (c) Refer for drug abuse treatment, as needed; (d) Provide psychosocial support systems; and (e) Provide a safe environment (i.e., inpatient care) where suicide can be prevented.

4. There may be phases of some individuals' career development where illness behaviors occur in adaptable forms. As illnesses change, however, or job responsibilities demand change during career development, illness behaviors can become maladaptive.

5. Ahlskog JE. *Dyskinesias*. Paper presented at: Parkinson's disease and movement disorders for the practitioner. Mayo Clinic, Scottsdale, Arizona, November 17–18, 1995.

6. Gold M, Adair JC, Jacobs DH, Heilman KM. Anosognosia for hemiplegia: an electrophysiologic investigation on the feed-forward hypothesis. *Neurology* 1994;44:1804–1808.

7. Andreasen NC. *The broken brain*. New York: Harper & Row; 1984:250.

8. Martin BA, Glancy GD. Consent to electroconvulsive therapy: investigation of the validity of a competency questionnaire. *Convulsive therapy* 1994;10:279–286.

9. Following is the three-step approach to competency determination from a medical standpoint:

   a. Establish the neurological functions necessary for being considered medically competent

b. Establish brain dysfunction that might interfere with the neurological functions required for medical competence
c. Determine the way in which brain dysfunction interferes with the neurological functions necessary for medical competence

The above guidelines also can be applied to competency to stand trial or assist a trial attorney.

4

Brain Failure

Like a fiend in a cloud,
With howling woe,
After night I do crowd,
And with night will go;
I turn my back to the east,
From whence comforts have increased;
For light doth seize my brain
With frantic pain.

William Blake
Poetical Sketches—Mad Song

Being possessed by illness behavior is hell. A patient cannot enjoy the
present, view the past or see the future.

Robert A. Williams, M.D.

At this point I would like to reiterate the purpose of this text. While its primary focus is to explain brain function and the role of biological psychiatry in restoring healthy function, there also is a secondary focus—to perpetuate a social movement based on true understanding about brain function. This understanding is an essential prerequisite for the effective treatment of brain failure in that it signifies acceptance of brain failure as a legitimate medical condition.

Part of acceptance of brain failure as a medical condition involves two beliefs:

1. Medical disorders that affect the brain are *not* disorders of will or self-control.
2. Medical disorders of the brain cause generators of behavior to produce behavior *independent of* (a) the physiological matrix of the personality, and (b) the present and past content of life.

Throughout the text I will use the terms "brain failure" and "psychosis" synonymously. As stated in Chapter 1, "psychosis" is defined in DSM-III-R as "gross impairment in reality testing and

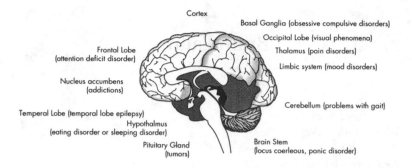

Cortex

Basal Ganglia (obsessive compulsive disorders)

Occipital Lobe (visual phenomena)

Frontal Lobe
(attention deficit disorder)

Thalamus (pain disorders)

Limbic system (mood disorders)

Nucleus accumbens
(addictions)

Cerebellum (problems with gait)

Temperal Lobe (temporal lobe epilepsy)

Hypothalmus
(eating disorder or sleeping disorder)

Pituitary Gland
(tumors)

Brain Stem
(locus coerleous, panic disorder)

The brain fails in its usual capacities

Figure 4-1. Brain model showing location of illness behavior.

the creation of a new reality."[1] Because "reality" is not rationally definable, however, I offer the following more operational definition of "psychosis": *any overt behavior that clearly represents brain dysfunction and impedes normal human functioning with regard to self and/or interpersonal, social or work relationships and activities.*

Brain failure, from a neuropsychiatric point of view, is failure of the normal brain capacities. The brain consists of multiple generators of behavior that create a physiological matrix we call personality.[2] Each generator of behavior operates within a window of physiological normalcy. If a given generator of behavior produces too much or too little activity, the abnormally functioning generator of behavior will produce different clinical syndromes (Fig. 4-1). In the case of very mild brain failure, if there is no disruption of human functioning, I define this as brain aberration (perhaps, the voice of conscience that speaks louder than usual).

Clinical Manifestations of Brain Failure

Brain failure is the result of either primary or genetic conditions and also may occur secondary to medical conditions, such as stroke, multiple sclerosis, brain tumor, hypothyroidism, head trauma, and a host of other conditions. The clinical presentations of brain failure are the *same* regardless of the cause.

When the brain fails in its usual capacities, predictable patterns are produced with illness, depending on the specific part of the brain that is affected. *All* brain failure can be identified by three clinical presentations, with the Mental Status Exam (MSE) serving as one of the principal identification tools:

1. **traditional psychosis** includes several broad areas of human function, such as language and perception dysfunction
2. **behavioral clusters** are characterized by relevant groups of signs and symptoms that predict brain failure
3. **specific lobe dysfunction** is caused by dysfunction in specific areas of the brain

Traditional psychosis represents the oldest means of identifying brain failure. Because it involves large areas of normal, visible functioning (language, belief, perception, and experience), traditional psychotic behavior appears abnormal, even to the casual observer. Areas of function typically are reflected in the following forms:

Thought disorder (reflected in language)
Scrambled or confused language reflects a psychotic thought process. For example, consider a patient (who is known to hear and speak without impairment) being questioned by a psychiatrist. If the patient understands specific queries but gives answers to other unrelated questions, this reflects a thought disorder and represents brain dysfunction. (The casual observer might comment: "He is talking 'crazy.'")[3]

Belief disorder (reflected in delusions)
Individuals who have a belief disorder typically manifest a dominant and persistent false mental belief of one of five major types (The casual observer might comment: "He has crazy beliefs."):[4]
Erotomanic type—characterized by belief that one is loved by another person, usually a public figure
Grandiose type—characterized by belief that one has a great, but unrecognized, talent or insight
Jealous type—characterized by belief that one's spouse or lover is unfaithful
Persecutory type—characterized by belief that one is being plotted against, followed, harassed, or unfairly prevented from accomplishing specific objectives.

Somatic type—characterized by belief that one is giving off a foul odor, that certain parts of the body are deformed, unattractive, or not functioning.

Perceptual disorder (reflected in hallucinations)

Individuals connect with the external world through the five senses: sight, smell, taste, touch, and hearing. When any of these modalities creates a false sensation (i.e., hearing voices or seeing people that don't exist), such hallucinations signal the presence of a perceptual disorder. (The casual observer might comment: "He is seeing crazy things.")

Experiential disorder (reflected in unusual experiences)

All individuals experience such normal emotions as love, hate, guilt, and fear, which are unrelated to beliefs. When there is a feeling that the body is being controlled like a robot, or that thoughts are "escaping" from the brain, an experiential disorder is present.[5] (The casual observer might comment: "He is having crazy experiences.")

Behavioral clusters represent *groups* of behavioral signs and symptoms that manifest at the same time and demonstrate the presence of brain failure. Most diagnoses in medicine involve identification of patterns and symptom clusters. For example, heart failure is clinically defined by a cluster of symptoms that includes an enlarged heart, shortness of breath, and ankle swelling.

Consider a man who enters his physician's office with a shuffling gait, tremor in his hands, muscle rigidity, and difficulty in initiating and ceasing movement; he has a *motor* behavioral cluster. It represents a basal ganglia dysfunction (failure in a particular part of the brain), and is caused by sick and dying brain cells that are producing decreased amounts of a specific neurotransmitter called dopamine. Although the man's behavior appears to give outward evidence of brain failure, mainline psychiatry would conclude that no *psychosis* is present, because symptoms reflect only motor behavioral abnormalities and not emotional difficulties.[6,7]

In DSM-IV behavioral clusters are described that (a) define brain failure (psychosis), and (b) relate to disruptions in human functioning. One common behavioral cluster that represents brain failure is major depression syndrome.[8] Major depression syndrome consists of at least a 2-week period when mood is depressed or irritable and an individual manifests at least five out of the nine following traits the majority of the time.

1. Depressed mood
2. Diminished interest in activities
3. Significant weight loss or gain
4. Insomnia or hypersomnia
5. Psychomotor agitation or retardation
6. Fatigue
7. Feelings of excessive guilt
8. Diminished ability to concentrate
9. Recurrent thoughts of death or suicide[9]

If a patient satisfies the DSM-IV criteria for major depression, then—by definition—the patient has brain failure. Again, behavioral clusters are determined by scientific and statistical methods. Therefore, if a patient can be characterized by a statistical cluster, there is a 96 percent chance that the cluster represents brain failure in that individual.[10] (Appendix D provides a case study of major depression syndrome.)

Specific lobe dysfunction, sometimes specified as a "neuro-psychiatric syndrome," occurs when there is failure of a well defined area, or lobe, of the brain that controls a particular function. A lesion in the frontal lobe, for example, might impair judgment, whereas an injury to the hippocampus of the temporal lobe might impair memory function. This third classification of brain failure is distinctly different from traditional psychosis (which relates to broad areas of brain function that are not localized) and behavioral clusters (which are derived empirically without reference to the location of brain dysfunction).

Specific lobe dysfunction can be caused by localized effects of stroke, tumor, aneurysm, trauma, and plaque formed by multiple sclerosis. Since different lobes of the brain have varying sensitivities to metabolic effects, specific lobe dysfunction can be caused by generalized metabolic problems, such as low oxygen, low vitamin levels, or low blood sugar.[11]

When specific lobe dysfunction is the cause of brain failure, the presence of specific lobe activation or inhibition deserves special consideration. In general, the brain is activated (or "turned on") by the Reticular Activating System (RAS) of the brain stem (lower brain). This level of consciousness, or wakefulness, can be viewed as brain (cortical) activation.

During sleep, the brain's cortex is deactivated ("turned off") and the midbrain takes over control of the various stages of sleep. During wakefulness, the RAS predominates and activates the cortex of the brain. In abnormal states, as seen in cases of head trauma, patients may experience reduced levels of activation, which may cause stuporous or coma-like states. A specific area of brain dysfunction may result in *global* brain dysfunction (where the brain is "turned off.")

Frontal lobe dysfunction is an example of specific lobe dysfunction and can be observed in many neuropsychiatric conditions; one example is Attention Deficit Disorder (ADD). ADD patients are unable to apply their knowledge, experience or intelligence because "working memory" in the frontal lobe is reduced. Because of frontal lobe dysfunction, ADD patients lack control over organization of time and executive functions.

The Cause and Effect of Abnormal Behavior

All dysfunctional human activity is not a result of psychosis/brain dysfunction. Since most behavior is genetically determined, statistical distribution of behavior can be observed. Some individuals with low IQs, for example, may exhibit abnormal cognitive ability, but show no signs of illness behavior. In these instances, low IQ is an expected behavior, as seen in a bell-shaped curve of IQ, and is not due to illness. On the other hand, there are many cases of lower-than-average intelligence, secondary to a medical illness, when low IQ occurs unexpectedly.

Society also plays a major role in shaping behavior through the teaching of social mores. If individuals mature in environments that teach or socialize clear principles of right and wrong, the physiology of the brain tends to keep those individuals on the "straight and narrow" path. There are two basic brain mechanisms that help people maintain social norms.

1. **Guilt or shame** (negative reinforcers): Guilt is produced by individuals who deviate from *learned* social norms, while shame is produced by other individuals directly *imposing* their values on others.
2. **Approval** (positive reinforcer): The sense of approval that comes from being watched and affirmed by others has a powerful effect on behavior. The sense of being judged is

closely related to being approved but can be another type of
negative reinforcer.

Most of us, in addition to responding to instinctive brain
mechanisms, are motivated to maintain social norms by the
thought of dealing with the law or going to prison. Some
unfortunates (sociopaths) do not have these instinctive capacities
nor the capability to learn to live within social norms. The form of
brain failure experienced by sociopaths renders them unable to
feel guilt or shame.

Clearly, social dysfunction is a complex issue only a portion of
which is caused by brain failure. There are many explanations for
antisocial activity. Certain segments of society may have
subcultural norms that are viewed as antisocial by other cultural
groups. The assassination attempt on President Ronald Reagan
was carried out, for example, by a radical who had been socialized
into believing he was doing something honorable. In some urban
ghetto environments, theft, extortion by intimidation, and
prostitution may be acceptable norms. Drug use and drug cultures
provide a foundation for a wide variety of antisocial behavior.
Drug use, alone, may limit the brain's capacity to observe socially
acceptable parameters. Drug cultures devalue social norms and
provide a cult standard, in the form of gangs, that supports
antisocial behavior.

One of the most notable impacts of abnormal behavior on
society is reflected financially. Just as individuals with low IQs
generally need special educational opportunities and costly social
support alternatives, individuals who manifest antisocial behavior
frequently require expensive, customized treatment and
programs, often including incarceration.

Abnormal behavior caused by brain failure also has a critical
effect on our society's mortality rate. Failure of any organ system in
the body, including the brain, can result in death. The death rate
linked to brain failure is appreciated by very few people, but
usually takes four primary forms:

Suicide

Individuals who become hopeless, depressed and suicidal are
motivated by an *illness*, not rational thought. In the United States
approximately 30,000 take their own lives each year. The cause of
death is not a "self-inflicted gunshot wound," as many death
certificates note; it is brain failure, i.e., behavior generated by
illness.

Accidents
Brain failure can cause faulty judgment, as well as decreased ability to concentrate or physically react. Such conditions can result in fatal auto accidents and often are responsible for serious falls at nursing homes.

Lack of motor activity
Particularly in old age, brain failure can block signals to stimulate physical movement while individuals are awake or asleep. The resulting inactivity can cause compression of the veins (phlebitis), formation of pulmonary embolisms, compression of skin and resulting infection, sepsis, lung compression (atelectasis), and pneumonia. Most nursing home patients die from brain failure, while many of the motivating factors that bring about nursing home placement also result from brain failure.

Malnutrition
Anorexia nervosa and other disorders can result in death because of inability or unwillingness to eat.

Abnormal behavior—whether or not it is a product of brain failure—demands greater emphasis on prevention and treatment research, from a biological perspective. Not only do its various forms present a massive economic burden for society, but immeasurable heartache for individuals and family members who are directly affected.[12]

Identifying Brain Failure

Brain failure, or psychosis, occurs when one or more generators of behavior leave the normal physiological matrix (personality) and create activity that is independent of normal feedback and regulatory mechanisms (i.e., independent of the behavior that governs personality). In such cases, independent generators of behavior—which may be caused by genetic or traumatic insult—interfere with normal brain capacity and produce illness (Fig. 4-2). It is important to note that the three clinical presentations of brain failure previously described—traditional psychosis, behavioral clusters, and specific lobe dysfunction—occur as a result of generators of behavior becoming independent of the personality matrix.

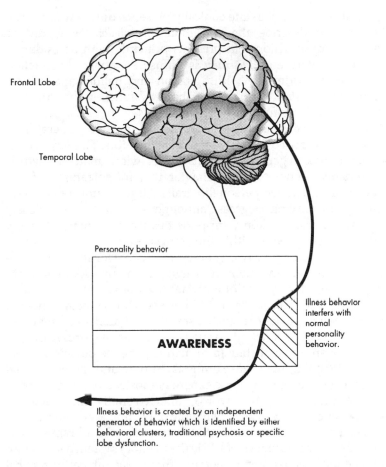

Frontal Lobe

Temporal Lobe

Personality behavior

AWARENESS

Illness behavior interfers with normal personality behavior.

Illness behavior is created by an independent generator of behavior which is identified by either behavioral clusters, traditional psychosis or specific lobe dysfunction.

Figure 4-2. The Williams Brain Model and identifying brain failure.

Factors that affect the metabolism of generators of behavior can cause brain failure or even death. Mild metabolic derangements can cause the more sensitive generators to fail differentially from other generators of behavior. For example, mild metabolic effects (i.e., anxiety and panic attacks) are seen with mild forms of hypoxia, such as chronic obstructive lung disease.

As metabolic dysfunction becomes more severe, a more overarching effect on brain generators occurs. Generalized metabolic dysfunction is called encephalopathy, delirium, or an acute confusional state. Depending on the way in which a generalized metabolic state clinically presents, different terms can be used to describe the condition. *Encephalopathy* is diffuse metabolic dysfunction that presents primarily with obtundation (decreased alertness). *Delirium* is diffuse metabolic dysfunction that presents primarily with agitation and hallucinations.[13] An *acute confusion state* is diffuse metabolic dysfunction that presents primarily with confusion and memory loss.

In a general sense, the brain is one massive generator of behavior comprised of many separate generators. This large series of superimposed generators forms the behavioral matrix known as personality. Generators of behavior that form features of our personality are called personality traits. All generators of behavior interact to varying degrees, although some are more closely associated. Brain anatomy supports this view, as there are many interconnecting loops within the brain substance.

An example of how two generators of behavior interact can be seen with anxiety and memory. There is a tendency for memory to improve in the presence of a certain level of anxiety. As anxiety increases, however, it begins to interfere with memory function. Finally, when anxiety reaches a severely agitated state, memory function ceases to function normally. Posttraumatic stress disorder (PTSD) is an unusual state (a human experience outside normal parameters) that may cause amnesia, in part, and memories that cause a graphic reliving of the experience instead of mere memory of the event. In other words, affected individuals actually reexperience events instead of having only unpleasant memories.

The behavior pattern of PTSD fits the model for brain failure. First, under the influence of PTSD the memory system becomes an independent generator of memory that is *not* subject to normal memory mechanisms. Normal initiators of memory are bypassed. In fact, the memory of an event may occur spontaneously or in response to an association. Second, the memory of an event is recorded abnormally. Under normal circumstances, individuals remember painful events but do not *reexperience* them. For example, a woman remembers the pain of childbirth (a normal experience) but does not relive the pain. PTSD patients, on the other hand, have intrusive memories that involve actually reexperiencing painful events.[14]

Coming into Awareness

Awareness, which has its center in the frontal lobes, is a well developed part of the human brain. Defined as "sustained reflective thought," awareness is comprised of the following elements:

1. Awareness of the thought itself
2. Awareness of the appropriateness of the thought, according to a specific situation
3. Awareness of the source of the thought (i.e., instinct vs. memory)
4. Belief awareness (i.e., is the thought true or not?)
5. Intensity of thought

For further details on awareness, refer to the box, "Understanding the Awareness Array," on page 62.

The process of awareness involves subjective assignments to sensory inputs, which can be divided into two categories: external to the brain and internal to the brain. The external world provides sensory inputs involving time, space, energy, and mass, and the brain provides subjective assignments in response to these elements. Subjective assignments then are directed to the awareness center, which create sustained reflective thoughts or a sense of awareness.[15]

Specific processes also may influence subjective assignments in the brain. Drugs, such as marijuana, can slow the sense of passing time. Seizures, such as those associated with temporal lobe epilepsy, may create visual images. Even emotional states, such as anxiety or impatience, affect subjective assignments.[16]

When all instinctive generators of behavior are satisfied, the awareness center is in a "free" state.[17] When instinctive generators of behavior (such as food, sex, or sleep) are not satisfied, instinctive generators of behavior activate a subjective assignment and provide specific obsessive thoughts within the awareness center. If instincts are not satisfied, the intensity of specific obsessive thoughts increases.

For example, fashion models, gymnasts, jockeys, and others who are required to be below their normal body weight usually are obsessed by thoughts of food. A genetically determined point within the hypothalamus sets body weight, and when individuals attempt to reduce their weight below 10 to 15 percent of the set point, there are very strong biological consequences.[18] The powerful instinctive "hunger" messages sent to the awareness center make it increasingly difficult for executive function to shift away from thoughts of food and a dysphoric mood state. Dreams begin to focus on hunger and eating. In a sense, executive function becomes "stuck" in one place until the instinctive generator of behavior is satisfied.

The life of models and others who self-impose strict diets and exercise programs can be seriously disrupted, in terms of interpersonal and social functioning. Although many envy the external beauty of models, the inner torment and suffering they experience is a heavy price to pay for being slender.

The internal world also is experienced in the frontal lobes of the brain. Generally, input to the frontal lobes travels from the brain stem up to the frontal lobes where individuals may become aware of instinctive behavior, if certain thresholds are exceeded.

The frontal lobes have executive function for directing brain activity and focusing awareness. Part of frontal lobe function is the use of working memory to synthesize time, resources, intelligence, creativity, and experience to reach goals.

Executive function, for example, can utilize working memory to solve problems. Problem-solving and the creative process then produce solutions that lead to productivity. Awareness is always a conscious process and only can occur when an individual is alert. Even during sleep, electroencephalographic analysis reveals alert or awake patterns during dream (REM) states (i.e., the individual who is sleeping must be in an alert state in order to be aware of dreams). Dream states are unique, however, because individuals in a dream state have the capacity to *experience* events, whereas individuals in an awake state normally only *remember* events.

Because the awareness center is such a highly developed part of the brain, it plays a major role in mental illness. As mentioned earlier, every input into the awareness center is the result of a unique subjective assignment, depending on the input. Sexual awareness and sense of body form are normal instincts. Patients with anorexia nervosa, a body form disorder, see themselves in a normal visual manner (visual pathways are intact) but routinely believe, perceive and experience awareness of themselves as overweight in spite of being grossly underweight. Brain failure, in this instance, selectively involves the part of the brain that relates to the subjective assignment, the sense of body form.

Brain failure may involve one or more generators of behavior. Depending on the sensitivity of a given generator of behavior to a specific physiological stressor, varying clinical syndromes are produced. For instance, hormonal stress (as seen in menopausal women) may manifest simply as intermittent autonomic hot flashes or as multiple symptoms of brain failure, such as insomnia, intestinal discomfort or increased appetite.

Some illnesses are partially defined by patients' awareness of their illness. For instance, the definition of obsessive compulsive disorder specifies that "the person recognizes that the obsessional thoughts, impulses or images are a product of his or her own mind."[19]

Other illnesses, such as mania, schizophrenia, psychotic depression, and addiction, typically include lack of awareness with other symptoms. Addiction, for example, is the creation of an independent generator that produces the desire or craving for a substance not normally required for life-sustaining needs. The addiction generator, for the most part, bypasses the awareness center. It is common for addicted individuals to be unable to see or be aware that their craving for a substance constitutes an illness.

Awareness of illness or perception of illness is a major factor in treating brain failure.[20] When a patient cannot perceive or believe that illness is present, then noncompliance follows. Resistance to treatment generally leads to frustration and feelings of helplessness among friends and family members. It is common to hear complaints, such as, "How can my son possibly get well? He doesn't even believe he has an illness."

In patients with manic disorders, the capacity to be aware of illness may be state-dependent. This means that when patients are in a normal mood state, they have normal awareness capacity. When patients are in a manic state, there may be no capacity for awareness of illness (either through perception or belief). In manic patients, even awareness of memories may be distorted. For example, awareness of memories that occurred during past manic episodes, especially resentment, may become activated in the awareness center.

The unfortunate consequences of lack of awareness in mental illness are many. These include:

1. mortality and morbidity
2. hospitalization
3. loss of job
4. divorce
5. severe stress on family and friends
6. antisocial behavior, often leading to imprisonment
7. loss of friends and social support systems
8. drug abuse
9. economic disaster
10. severe personal stress
11. repercussions stemming from inaccurate diagnosis[21]

As mentioned before, many conditions may manifest as traditional psychosis. Part of the psychotic process involves intrusive thoughts within the awareness center. For example, paranoid patients who become cognizant of their behavior created by brain dysfunction may be acutely aware of their suspiciousness or fear of harm by others. At the same time they are unaware of the *source* of suspiciousness, that it is a product of the brain.

Psychotic processes activate the same subjective assignments that would have been activated in the presence of actual threatening sensory inputs. Psychotic patients are aware and experience threats to their existence. This occurs in sharp contrast to hypomanic patients whose behavior may circumvent awareness. Acute paranoid schizophrenic patients experience fears and intrusive paranoid thoughts that dominate their awareness, but they have no capacity to see the source of their thoughts.

Panic anxiety disorder provides a good illustration of the role awareness plays in illness. During a panic attack patients are aware of and experience a sense of impending doom, but because the attack typically lasts only a few minutes, this sensation is short-lived. After the attack, the patient immediately recognizes that the subjective assignments relating to death were part of the panic attack and not real.

Even though panic patients may feel normal between attacks and may have experienced dozens of them, during the attack itself they never develop the capacity to "see" it as anything but real. The impact of panic attacks is severe, much like being randomly hit over the head with a two-by-four. In fact, 20 percent of panic patients commit suicide.

The panic attack is an example of a short-term "psychosis." Awareness of the symptoms is prominent and the subjective assignments are "real," both of which block insight or awareness of the true source of symptoms.

Awareness: The Pathway to Wellness

It is important to note that activation of subjective assignments to sensory inputs produces phenomena that are experienced as though they were real.

Acceptance of brain failure generally involves three neurological functions:

1. the capacity to "see," perceive, or experience a problem
2. the capacity to crystallize a belief (a highly socially determined process) about the problem[22]
3. the capacity to act on belief

In most instances, affected individuals are prone to "deny" the presence of their own illness. At every turn there is a cognitive choice to ignore memories of the actual illness experience, to turn away from learned information about the illness and to cognitively disavow beliefs about the illness.[23]

With mental illness we have all the normal mechanisms that prevent acceptance of illness and some unique ones as well. As discussed previously, the most notable feature of mental illness that prevents acceptance is patients' incapacity to "see" their illness. If individuals are unaware of their illness, they are not likely to accept its existence.[24] A second notable feature about mental illness is the social stigma of the disease itself. Because mental illness is so poorly understood, public attitude toward it is very negative and frequently is illustrated when affected individuals are prevented from participating in activities with unaffected individuals (the "blackball effect.")

A key step in treating brain failure, therefore, lies in creating an environment where patients can become aware of their illness. This can be done in several ways:

Patients can experience consequences of their behavior
Despite their inability to "see" their own abnormal behavior, patients *can* recognize that family members are angry or that friends no longer want to socialize with them. Psychotherapy may help patients connect these consequences with behavior they cannot see. When family members are encouraged to exercise "tough love," for example, patients have an opportunity to see the consequences of their behavior.

Patients can recognize their illness, based on the faith they have in friends, family members or religious leaders
This is made possible by the spiritual part of the brain that allows for belief (such as a belief in God) in things that are unseen.

Patients can be encouraged
Patients can be encouraged by groups of family members or friends who create a safe support system, or social matrix, that facilitates belief in and acceptance of illness.

Patients who have the capacity for awareness can be taught through their awareness center to differentiate between normal behavior and behavior generated by illness.[25] The first principle I present to my patients is that their behavior is created by illness that exists *independent* of their personality and apart from the present and past content of their lives.[26] Many patients ask, "What else is there?" and my response is similar to the multiple-question test answer, "None of the above." *Behavior generated by brain failure frequently causes intrusive thoughts that are completely unrelated to past or present experience. Illness behavior enters the awareness center and compromises normal brain capacity.*

Approximately 75 percent of psychiatric patients can be taught to monitor the presence of psychiatric illness in their awareness center. (See Appendix E for case study of a patient who effectively uses self-monitoring technique.) This can be done in the same way an asthmatic is taught to monitor lung function or a diabetic is taught to measure blood sugar levels. The awareness center can be monitored in the following ways to detect evidence of brain failure:

1. Monitor awareness of illness symptoms manifested in illness behavior (internal awareness) or consequences of behavior (external awareness)[27]
2. Remain sensitive to emotional overreactivity, decreased capacity to cope with stress, or suicidal thoughts that may affect interpersonal and social behavior, i.e., awareness of emotional instability[28]
3. Watch for decreased capacity to function (seen in severe depression) that may affect industrial functioning, i.e., awareness that cognitive functioning is compromised

For particularly insightful and motivated patients who lack internal awareness of their illness, external awareness or consequences of illness can be used to monitor the presence of illness. Some hypomanic patients, for instance, who cannot perceive their own mania, still can note the presence of illness by watching for elevated mood, racing thoughts, decreased need for sleep, increased capacity for pleasure, increased spending, sudden outbursts of anger, interpersonal and work-related problems.

Schizophrenic patients may "see" only the *obsessive* nature of their illness as being abnormal. Therapy is directed at the repeated intrusive behavior that schizophrenic patients may recognize as abnormal. Suspicious thoughts and delusions typically are seen and experienced as normal and, therefore, cannot be used for self-monitoring.

When patients understand more about their behavior caused by brain failure, they are better equipped to direct and accept therapy.[29] By monitoring their own illness, learning to modify awareness (when possible), and using medication within specific guidelines (based on physiological needs of the illness), patients are able to develop a sense of independence. (See "Understanding the Awareness Array" on page 62.) Self-monitoring enhances coping skills and facilitates strong cognitive responses, which significantly reinforces the effects of medication:

- "I can identify my illness."
- "I can do something about my illness."
- "I can control my illness."

Prevailing public attitude creates the matrix that dictates our society's beliefs about brain failure. Currently, social guidelines support psychological and social determinants of behavior despite a growing trend in support of biological determinants. Because the capacity to change the existing belief system varies broadly and because belief system stress is so widespread throughout our western culture, it might be well to consider implementing a social education program to address this issue in the United States. Currently, our nation is experiencing the "Decade of the Brain," a period mandated by the United States Congress to educate the public about the brain. Needless to say, efforts thus far have been inadequate and have focused mainly on the neurology of the brain.

Although it may be difficult, psychiatric treatment of brain failure can offer patients several avenues for social acceptance:

1. Referral to support groups that promote education and counter social stigma
2. Referral to educational materials
3. Referral for supportive psychotherapy
4. Referral to this text, *Brain Basics*, for clarification of brain function and failure

In conclusion, awareness is a sustained reflective thought. Through executive function, individuals can direct inputs, such as memories, into awareness and control brain function. Or, instincts

Understanding the Awareness Array

The awareness center is comprised of an array of awareness cells (levels of awareness). Each cell is responsible for a specific area of awareness, which receives unique subjective assignments related to unique functions. These areas range from the most basic sensory inputs to sophisticated spiritual and creative components. Awareness progresses, or shifts, from one awareness cell to the next.

Following is an example of how awareness progresses from the most basic sensory input to the more advanced capacities for creativity and dramatic expression:

1. The internal sense focuses on feeling, or being aware of, the left wrist
2. The external sense focuses on the silence or noise in a room
3. Instinct poses questions about the presence of hunger or the need for sleep
4. Memory focuses on recalling the first day of kindergarten
5. Working memory can visualize an eagle soaring in the sky
6. The sense of self focuses on personal feelings
7. Spirituality focuses on the presence of divine forces or a divine creator outside oneself
8. The social sense focuses on how the self is perceived by others
9. Obsessiveness formulates and executes plans for the future
10. Creativity forms new ideas and concepts for poetic verse
11. Initiation of a motor task can focus on miming (or pretending to execute) a specific activity, such as hammering a nail into a wall

When an individual allows his or her executive function to guide the awareness shift, it is called *self-generated* (self-hypnosis). When someone else guides the shift, it is called *hypnosis*.

Understanding awareness is a key factor in monitoring the presence of illness behavior for two primary reasons:

1. Illness behavior *may* intersect awareness and provide a basis for tracking the effects of medication and/or maintenance therapy.
2. Illness behavior that *does* intersect awareness is based on a particular generator of behavior that is dysfunctional.

Following is a list of the various awareness cells and examples of associated illness behaviors that can result in the presence of independent generators of behavior.

Awareness Cell	Illness Behavior
Sensory input (internal)	Auditory hallucinations
Sensory input (external)	Suspicion about the behavior of others
Instinct	Eating disorder
Memory	Alzheimer's disease
Working memory	Attention deficit disorder
Sense of self	Mood disorder
Spirituality	Lack of awareness of or inability to feel spirituality
Social sense	Social phobia
Obsessiveness	Obsessive compulsive disorder
Creativity	Lack of creativity
Initiation of complex motor tasks	Parkinson's disease

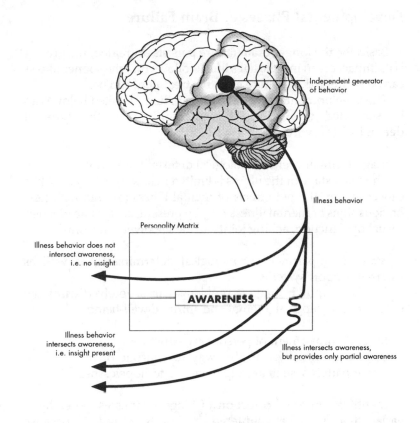

Independent generator
of behavior

Illness behavior

Personality Matrix

Illness behavior does not
intersect awareness,
i.e. no insight

AWARENESS

Illness behavior
intersects awareness,
i.e. insight present

Illness intersects awareness,
but provides only partial awareness

Figure 4-3. Williams Brain Model and awareness.

can directly intrude on awareness. Mental illness (i.e., independent generators of behavior) can interact with awareness in several ways (Fig. 4-3) by:

1. Completely bypassing awareness, as seen in addiction and hypomania
2. Intersecting awareness with awareness that the behavior is abnormal, as seen in obsessive-compulsive disorder
3. Intersecting awareness without awareness that the behavior is abnormal, as seen in schizophrenia and panic disorder

Clearly, awareness is a significant behavioral determinant, and its role as such will be discussed in greater detail in Chapter 5.

Developmental Phases of Brain Failure

Basically, the longer brain failure persists untreated, the greater is its impact on an individual's life. It follows that the sooner illness can be addressed, the more effective treatment can be.

The developmental phases of brain failure (detailed below) can be separated into three stages, according to the type of determinants involved.

Stage 1: Impairment of biological determinants only

The acute stage of the illness is limited in its scope. If treated like cancer in situ, the net effects of mental illness are minimal. Less obvious signs of mental illness may be present, such as headaches, sexual dysfunction, aching joints, irritable bowel syndrome.

Stage 2: Impairment of biological determinants, as well as external support systems

Left unattended, Stage 2 problems can severely disrupt the sense of psychological, mental and spiritual well-being.

Stage 3: Impairment of personality structure

Stage 3 eventually can give way to neurotic or maladaptive behavior patterns, such as helplessness and hopelessness.

Identification and correction of Stage 1 illnesses generally is easier than those encountered in Stages 2 and 3, because psychological and social impacts are greatest and most varied during later stages. Stress management (which will be discussed at greater length in Chapter 10) can be beneficial at all levels, but especially during Stage 1, when stress factors can be linked directly to specific biological problems. The primary types of stress that can lead to brain failure include: (a) background stressors that are a natural part of an individual's social status, family role, etc.; (b) chronic stressors that are part of daily life (financial strain, professional or academic performance, overcommitment, etc.); (c) life-change stressors that upset the normal pattern of living (illness, new job, financial reversal, etc.); (d) traumatic stressors that usually happen infrequently but have long-lasting effects (birth, marriage, death, divorce, relocation, etc.).[30]

Two other types of stress, which are based primarily on fear, often are seen in the later stages of brain failure. First, if individuals are aware of the consequences of mental illness, that recognition (if not monitored appropriately) can have powerfully demoralizing effects. Anxiety over other people's perceptions of mental illness, together with poor self-image and low self-esteem, can make rehabilitation very challenging. Lack of support from family and friends who may be frustrated, confused and angered by the symptoms of brain failure can further compound the difficulties.

Second, fear of being possessed by irrational independent behaviors that are *not* part of will or self-control can be overwhelming for many patients. Education can be invaluable when it emphasizes the importance of maintaining (a) internal awareness to identify illness, and (b) flexibility to change doses of medication in response to active illness. When patients can retain a sense of control and a positive cognitive set of behaviors in response to active illness, they can cope more reasonably with normal fears of illness and can approach wellness with confidence. Fear of not getting well is almost always followed by the fear of not *staying* well.

Major Syndromes of Brain Failure

The brain can fail in any of its usual capacities. Since the brain has a large array of capacities, the brain can produce a vast assortment of syndromes. These syndromes traditionally are identified by their dominant or more obvious symptom. For instance, a major depressive syndrome is most noted for the presence of depressed mood, although other signs and symptoms are present.[31]

Scientists have determined from family studies and DNA analysis that a large number of psychiatric disorders have a major genetic determinant. Other psychiatric disorders have a major secondary determinant, such as strokes, multiple sclerosis, drugs, trauma, infection, and tumors. Some psychiatric disorders are probably the combination of genetic and environmental influences. All psychiatric disorders have the capacity to become generalized, affecting the entire brain. Ultimately, brain dysfunction can become diffuse and lead to catatonia.

As areas of failure spread, dysfunction increases until the entire brain can be affected. All diseases of the brain can potentially affect *any* generator of behavior. A disorder may begin with simple anxiety, move to agitation, depression, delirium, coma, and even death.

While psychiatrists treat many different types of brain disorders, four major categories of illness usually are considered to be most important and are linked to biological causes. Together, they affect millions of individuals and account for an incredible amount of human suffering.[32]

Affective disorders, which include manic and depressive disorders, are characterized by disturbances in affect or the way individuals cyclically experience mood. These events tend to occur episodically. Individuals with normal affect react to events with appropriate levels of happiness or sadness, whereas patients with affective disorders experience exaggerated levels of elation or unhappiness that are independent of personality.

It is believed that the limbic lobe regulates mood. Therefore, a chemical imbalance within the limbic lobe creates mood swings. Normally, the limbic lobe functions within limits that reflect the content of our lives, i.e., "good" days vs. "bad" days. With limbic system failure, behavior is generated that is independent of normal moods. Overactivity of the limbic system produces mania, while underactivity produces depression.

As noted earlier, the classic behavioral cluster for depression includes despair, hopelessness, insomnia, decreased appetite, social withdrawal, difficulty in concentrating, and loss of confidence. Suicide affects approximately 15 percent of all those hospitalized with depression.

Individuals with manic disorder appear to have endless energy and enthusiasm; however, their behavior also is marked by irritability, poor judgment, disorganized thought patterns, inflated self-esteem, and lapses into depression. Manics can get themselves and others into significant trouble as a result of their cavalier spending habits, poor business investments, impulsive decision-making, and antisocial behavior (i.e., public nudity).

Schizophrenic disorders tend to be noncyclical, chronically incapacitating, and affect roughly 1 person in every 100. Some forms of schizophrenia are marked by hallucinations and delusions, others by disturbed thinking and unusual emotional responsiveness. Typically, schizophrenic disorders are more difficult to understand than affective disorders. Schizophrenia is characterized by one or more of the traditional psychoses without associated symptoms of mood, anxiety or symptoms of other mental illness (i.e., an isolated psychosis without known cause, such as an LSD psychosis). Basically, schizophrenia is viewed as a heterogeneous disorder because of its varied presentations of psychosis.

Anxiety disorders, like affective disorders, occur with comparative frequency and are marked by the following physical and psychological symptoms that occur during a definite period of time: rapid pulse, pounding heart, chest pain, sweating, nausea, diarrhea, tension nervousness, and subjective feelings of panic.

Anxiety disorders manifest as a result of the brain's level of alertness or readiness. An overalert brain is characterized as "anxious." An underalert brain is characterized as "sedate." The Reticular Activating System in the brain stem is believed to be the generator of behavior that activates the cortex of the brain. As the brain is activated, individuals proceed through the following stages of anxiety:

1. mild subjective feeling of "edginess"
2. frank, or obvious, anxiety
3. agitation; a feeling of wanting to "jump out of (one's) skin;" motor overflow (wringing of the hands, pacing)
4. aggression manifested in self-destructive and/or overtly hostile acts, i.e., pounding on walls, throwing furniture, burning or cutting oneself

Anxiety disorders can be divided into three main subcategories (according to the DSM-IV):

Phobic disorders are characterized by continuous and irrational fear of a specific stimulus, leading to a persistent wish to avoid the source of fear Fear of being alone, or public speaking and heights are in this category.

Anxiety states are characterized by irrational fear that is unconnected to any particular stimulus.

- Panic disorder is marked by sudden and recurring attacks of anxiety.
- Generalized anxiety disorder is marked by persistent anxiety without phobias or panic attacks.
- Obsessive compulsive disorder is marked by a compulsion to complete a senseless, repetitive act, such as hand-washing or mirror-checking.

Posttraumatic stress disorders usually become evident following the occurrence of a traumatic stressor, such as participation in active combat or being held as a prisoner-of-war. Individuals with this condition feel as though they are reliving the negative experience and often report loss of ability to enjoy any life experience. Loss of all emotional response may be noted, along with difficulty in sleeping and hyperalertness.

Dementia is characterized by loss of cognitive function, usually starting with memory disturbance and progressing to psychosis. It is characterized by loss of intellectual capacity (especially memory) and emotional function, impaired social judgment, and gross personality changes. Alzheimer's disease is the most widely recognized condition in this category.

Specific types of brain failure are discussed more fully in chapters 6 and 7.

Summary

As the brain fails in its usual capacities, patients manifest a range of symptoms, depending on the specific generators of behavior that are involved.

The brain consists of multiple generators of behavior that form a physiological matrix called personality. Illness occurs when one or more generators of behavior become independent of the personality matrix and interfere with normal functioning.

All brain failure can be characterized by:

1. Behavioral clusters
2. Traditional psychosis
3. Specific lobe dysfunction

Special problems exist in treating individuals for mental illness:

1. Brain failure circumvents the capacity for awareness of abnormal behavior
2. Lack of social matrix (socialization) inhibits belief crystallization
3. Lack of education blocks understanding of brain basics and mental illness
4. Social stigma prohibits admission of brain failure symptoms

As patients understand brain basics, patients' capacity to control illness increases and can be implemented by following four primary steps:

1. Identify active symptoms of illness within the awareness center
2. Undestand that the source of behavior is biological, not content of life or personality

3. Direct biological therapy to control illness
4. Maintain strong cognitive set of behaviors that relate to independence and control over illness

Treatment success is most likely when the following elements are present:

1. Functional awareness of behavior that represents illness, i.e., independent generators of behavior
2. Understanding of the consequences of illness
3. Knowledge about behavior and illness
4. Understanding of the psychological and social consequences of illness
5. Experience with medication, crystallizing a belief about illness that leads to acceptance and rational treatment

In order to undergo treatment for brain failure, affected individuals must be aware of their condition. Although brain failure often obscures this awareness, some patients can learn to recognize thoughts and actions that are generated independent of normal personality and seek professional assistance when these traits develop.

Brain failure, which is governed by brain physiology and dictates the form of behavior, is the target of biological therapies. When a generator of behavior becomes independent of the personality structure and interferes with functioning, illness behavior is produced.

The psychology of the brain is a reflection of the content of behavior and is treated by psychological therapies. When a generator of behavior within the personality structure becomes maladaptive, neurotic behavior results.

Brain failure disorders are grouped into four main categories: (a) affective, (b) schizophrenic, (c) anxiety-related, and (d) dementia. Diseases of the brain are identified primarily by the most pronounced symptoms, although many generators of behavior can be affected and may produce countless symptoms.

Brain failure also may be classified according to chronicity:

1. Stage 1: Acute, not chronic
2. Stage 2: Psychological and social
3. Stage 3: Chronic, affecting personality structure
             (learned behavior)

References

1. *Diagnostic and statistical manual of mental disorders.* 3rd edition. Washington, DC: The American Psychiatric Association; 1987:404.
2. A generator of behavior is a system of neurons that has a common function, such as memory, language or mood regulation.
3. In our society the use of the term "crazy" is common. In some cases, the casual observer of an individual with brain failure might appropriately note "irrational" behavior and describe it as "crazy." Unfortunately, "crazy" has come to have a derogatory meaning. As we develop a better understanding of the brain, I hope that more humanistic principles will be applied and that "brain failure" will be used in place of "crazy."
4. *Diagnostic and statistical manual of mental disorders.* 4th edition. Washington, DC: The American Psychiatric Association; 1994:297–298.
5. At one time, experiential disorders were called "first rank symptoms," because first rank symptoms were thought to be specific (first rank) for schizophrenia. Now it is known that first rank symptoms occur in many psychiatric disorders, such as mania and organic psychosis.
6. The brain controls the following areas of function:

Robotics	Coordinated movement
Cognition	Thought
Emotions	Mood, affectivity
Reproduction	
Maintenance of	Monitoring of metabolic processes, internal homeostasis such as digestion, respiration, etc.

   Although dysfunction in the above-named areas represents brain failure in the strictest sense, "psychosis" generally is used to describe types of brain failure that directly contribute to humanistic behavior, that is behavior relating to the self and/or interpersonal, social and work relationships, and activities. While the psychiatrist specializes in treatment of brain failure that affects personal human experience (psychosis), the neurologist focuses on robotics, the internist focuses on issues of internal homeostasis and the reproductive specialist focuses on reproductive disorders.
7. I disagree with the artificial division of brain failure into categories, such as motor or emotional classifications. Brain failure is brain failure.
8. "Syndrome" is defined as organ system failure that has an unknown or undetermined cause.
9. These nine criteria, which are discussed on page 327 of DSM-IV, represent behavior (generated by the limbic system in the brain) that is independent of personality and independent of the content of an individual's life. Depressive thoughts created by the illness generator

are *not* the thoughts of the individual; rather, they intrude upon the awareness center from an independent source.

10. It is important to note that "brain failure" is not a diagnosis, because all brain failure presents in the same way from a clinical standpoint. Once the presence of brain failure has been determined, then the cause of brain failure can be sought. DSM-IV criteria only define brain failure; they do not define illness.

11. Following are three types of frontal lobe syndromes and examples of brain failure that each may cause:

   • orbital frontal
   • obsessive compulsive disorder
   • anterior cingulate
   • schizophrenia
   • dorsal lateral prefrontal
   • mood disorder

12. The economic cost of depression in the United States in 1990 equaled $43 billion. *Primary care update: clinical controversies in depression.* Santa Ana. CME, Inc.; November 1995:3.

13. David Conn explains in "Delirium and Other Organic Mental Disorders," that delirium—to which the elderly are particularly susceptible—has many causes, including environmental toxins, infections, low blood sugar, low vitamin levels, low oxygen, severe sleep deprivation, cerebral hemorrhage, and exposure to insecticides. (In: Sadavoy J, Lazarus L, Jarvik L, eds. *Comprehensive review of geriatric psychiatry.* Washington, DC: American Psychiatric Press, Inc.; 1991:313.)

14. Multiple personality disorder, which has been diagnosed in some children, truly is a form of PTSD. A growing number of psychiatric professionals believe that PTSD in children may cause disassociative disorder, which is characterized by the assumption of secondary personalities in order to avoid reexperiencing painful events. This cognitive adaptation to PTSD creates a multipersonality syndrome.

15. All of us have similar subjective assignments that allow us to share experiences and provide a basis for social existence. For instance, sense of time is experienced in the same way by all individuals, just as the colors of a rainbow are experienced in a similar fashion.

   We may perceive experiences in vastly different ways as well, as is the case with artistic appreciation. For example, centuries ago Greek and Roman artisans discovered the meaning of subjective assignments and awareness in their artwork. They assumed that a three- dimensional object, such as a statue, was necessary to produce a three-dimensional perception; they believed that a two-dimensional object, such as a painting, would produce a two-dimensional awareness. During the Renaissance, however, it was discovered that a two-dimensional painting could induce a three-dimensional perception or subjective assignment (i.e., illusion).

Through the years artists have experimented with a range of mediums to produce different subjective awareness. For instance, abstract art typically includes color and form that induces a subjective experience devoid of social or memory overlay. Impressionistic art utilizes abstraction and realism to produce yet another type of awareness. In summary, artists create works that produce a unique awareness that emanates from subjective experience.

16. In boring or awkward situations, it is fairly common for individuals to have the sense that time is virtually "standing still."
17. I define "free" as a state in which the frontal lobes are allowed to choose what they want to be aware of or think about.
18. This is the reason most diet programs eventually fail.
19. *Diagnostic and statistical manual of mental disorders.* 4th edition. Washington, DC: The American Psychiatric Association; 1994:423.
20. *Psychiatric Annals*, vol. 27, number 12 (December, 1997):782–811.
21. Mental illness patients may be inaccurately diagnosed as being in a state of "denial." The term, "denial," implies a psychological process but is inappropriate when real physical incapacities prevent patients from "seeing" their illness. Where there is no active perception, not only is it impossible for patients to see their illness but they have no capacity to believe they *have* an illness.
22. A belief is a memory that is categorized as either true or untrue. It is not known how a memory is crystallized into a belief or belief system. Certainly, the social matrix in which an individual lives influences beliefs.

    Cognitive therapists refer to "core beliefs," or the basic beliefs individuals have about themselves. Childhood trauma and abuse can lead to core beliefs that are negative, such as low self-esteem, lack of confidence, and self-blame. The crystallization of negative beliefs during childhood becomes part of the personality matrix (i.e., core beliefs). During adulthood negative core beliefs can result in maladaptive behavior.

    The following situation, describing the way in which an inappropriate belief (i.e., "I'm a bad person.") can crystallize in the wake of childhood abuse, illustrates the "ABC's" of cognitive behavior:

    A (Action): An individual may experience a normal stressor in life, such as doing poorly in school.

    B (Beliefs): Instead of responding to the stressor in a positive, constructive (adaptive) way (i.e., "I'll get tutored," or "I'll study more," or I'll talk with my teacher," the individual automatically adopts negative beliefs (i.e., I'm a bad person, and I can't do it.)

    C (Consequences): The result of automatic negative thoughts includes depression, hopelessness and helplessness (demoralization).

Each part of the above cognitive model of behavior involves different parts of the awareness array:

1. Perceptual awareness: Did poorly in school
2. Belief awareness: "I'm a bad person."
3. Self-awareness: Depression

The idea of cognitive therapy is to challenge and change core beliefs or automatic negative thoughts. Awareness is a major feature of cognitive therapy.

23. For example, 50 percent of adolescents under treatment for seizure disorders do not take their medications. Only a series of traumatic events (i.e., serious physical injury, social embarrassment, loss of driver's license) typically will move patients of this age to accept their illness.

24. Intellectual capacities, which exist independent of psychosis, are located in specific areas of the brain. In a society like ours where high intellectual level frequently can mask psychosis, it may be assumed that individuals who perform well intellectually cannot be psychotic. Nothing could be further from the truth. The tragedy of this assumption, however, regularly is played out within the legal system when apparently bright defendants are permitted to provide their own defense because they are experienced in legal proceedings. Psychotic patients who have no awareness of their illness will not file an insanity plea and may be completely incapable of organizing a rational defense.

   Because many neuropsychiatric disorders bypass awareness and individuals are legally protected from forced treatment, severe consequences of illness frequently are endured. The consequences include death, injury, legal problems, divorce, posttraumatic stress for loved ones and many others. If all efforts, including guidance and support from therapists, friends, family members and a knowledge of brain basics, cannot persuade a patient to seek medical help, legal measures (such as formal commitment to a medical facility) may be necessary. Unfortunately, many patients are in limbo in that they cannot be committed nor are they cooperative with treatment.

25. Patients can learn to discern between internal and external sensory input, can allow thoughts and emotions to occur simultaneously, and can learn to process multiple inputs.

26. Patients frequently comment, "No one understands me. My parents tell me I'm beautiful, intelligent and have everything to live for, but it doesn't help." It is common for parents and other concerned individuals to direct their support to the components of an individual's personality, but this approach has no impact in the case of brain failure. This is because illness-based behavior is *independent* of personality and content of life.

When I speak to a patient, I emphasize the following concepts:
- "I am not talking to you; I am talking to the behavior you are exhibiting that represents illness."
- "Your illness behavior has nothing to do with the content of your life."
- "Your behavior has nothing to do with your will or self-control."
- "There is nothing I can say that will change your behavior. Medical therapies are needed to change the physiology of your brain that has created this independent source of behavior."

27. Internal awareness depends on the generators of behavior that have failed. For instance, if the limbic system fails and results in a depressive behavioral cluster, the patient will be aware of depressed mood, decreased capacity to enjoy activities, slowed thinking, and other symptoms. If there is basal ganglial-frontal lobe failure resulting in obsessive compulsive disorder cluster, the patient will be aware of repetitive intrusion of unwanted thoughts.

28. When suicidal thoughts arise, I coach my patients to do the following:

- Say aloud, "My suicidal thoughts are not my thoughts. They are the thoughts of my illness."
- Remind yourself, "I want to get well. If I kill myself, I cannot get well."
- Remember to breathe deeply, slowly and fully. Take prescribed medications.

29. Great care must be taken by patients who initiate education about brain basics to process the significant conflicts that may arise between old and new behavioral attitudes. This conflict, known as "belief system stress," should be processed with the aid of a therapist or support group. Following is an example of the impact this type of stress can have on interpersonal relationships:

A husband and wife saw me in consultation for education with regard to the wife's depression. During our visit, the husband appeared intelligent and cooperative but, evidently, the information presented about brain physiology and its effect on behavior was too foreign for him to accept. Later, he became so angry and frustrated with his wife that he separated from her.

One evening while the husband was watching television, he heard an explanation of depression similar to the one I had presented to him and his wife. Finally, he was able to "accept/believe" depression as a type of brain failure, more than something "in her head," and returned to his wife soon thereafter.

30. Henn FA. Epidemiology of psychiatric illness. In: Winokur G, Clayton P, eds. *The medical basis of psychiatry*. Philadelphia: W B Saunders Co; 1986:554.

31. The evolution of nomenclature of psychiatric disorders reflects the more obvious symptom in a behavioral cluster, such as depression. As

more scientific and systematic studies are performed to evaluate major depressive syndromes, it has been found that 50 percent of patients with a major depressive syndrome are not depressed. Patients might feel irritable or anxious or dysmorphic but not depressed. They may experience slowed thinking, low motivation, sleep disturbance, low sex drive, decreased appetite, or suicidal thoughts, without depression. In fact, some psychiatric syndromes reflect misnomers but cannot be changed because the syndrome name is already well established in scientific literature. For instance, major depression would be more appropriately categorized as "psychomotor (mind and body) slowing."

32. Andreasen NC. *The broken brain.* New York: Harper & Row; 1984: 34–82.

5
Determinants of Behavior: An Open Model

From the moment of his birth the customs into which [an individual] is born shape his experience and behavior. By the time he can talk, he is the little creature of his culture.

Ruth Fulton Benedict
Patterns of Culture

The capacity to perceive and believe is a form of behavior that is genetically determined. What we see and believe—the content of behavior—is our culture.

Robert A. Williams, M.D.

The medical model, as we learned in Chapter 1, is a scientific and rational approach to medicine. This scientific framework is an essential tool in understanding brain physiology, although the complexities of human behavior transcend current capacities of science. The open model, an expansion of the medical model, is a method of considering all determinants of behavior, or factors that have an influence on behavior. Identification of specific behavioral determinants is important because it can lead to enhanced appreciation for underlying causes of brain failure (or maladaptive behavior) and the application of appropriate therapies.

The process of identifying determinants of behavior must be based on the neuropsychiatric brain model (henceforth referred to here as the *Williams Brain Model*), which is defined by the structure and arrangement of neurons and their electrochemical properties. Any process that disrupts the structure of the brain or the functioning neuron and, thus, has an impact on generators of behavior, may change overt behavior.

A Biological Overview

The protected environment of the womb serves to insulate the developing fetus from the outside world so neuronal structure/arrangement can be formed with minimal environmental influence. Unfortunately, purely functional development is not always possible as maternal infections, poor nutrition, drug use, and physical trauma can interrupt genetic expressions. Brain damage during the birth process also can cause varying levels of dysfunction (i.e., cerebral palsy). Any genetic defect or mutation may manifest itself during fetal development, which can be the cause of illness at birth or later in life.

Following birth, other determinants, which fall into three distinct but related categories, play an increasing role in determining behavior (Fig. 5-1). Biological foundations, which create brain structure and functioning neurons (form), are joined by psychosocial foundations (comprising content of life that shapes behavior) and spiritual foundations (making up the essence of life).

Several other variables can modify brain physiology—the genetic timeline, the aging process, memory formation, the educational process (both academic and social), and gestalt-type experiences.[1] Normally, these factors do not create illness behavior but may bring about personality changes.

When the brain fails in its usual capacities, brain failure manifests symptoms based on the specific area of the brain that fails.[2] A discussion about behavioral determinants can be confusing, however, because the brain fails in its usual capacities and produces the same symptoms, *regardless of the cause*. The DSM-IV criteria for major depression[3] reads, "The symptoms (of major depression) are not better accounted for by bereavement . . . ". This statement recognizes that the symptoms of bereavement (content of life related to loss) are similar to major depression.

Chapter 3 describes behavior in terms of form and content. In general, form is dictated by the physiology of the brain and content is determined by the content of life. Medical disorders that affect the brain have physiological determinants. Psychological disorders that affect the brain have content-of-life determinants. Spiritual disorders that affect the brain have spiritual content-of-life determinants.

The Williams Brain Model describes illness behavior as being comprised of independent generators of behavior that interfere

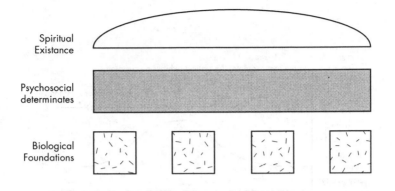

Spiritual
Existance

Psychosocial
determinates

Biological
Foundations

Figure 5-1. Hierarchy of behavior.

with normal human functioning. The stress model (Fig. 5-2) illustrates the way stress can affect the form of behavior.

Remember, form of behavior is determined by brain physiology. Normally, content of life affects only the psychology of behavior. Indirectly, life content in the form of stress can affect the form of behavior by decreasing the threshold for illness. When the threshold for illness intersects a generator of behavior, illness behavior results.

For example, epileptic patients traditionally experience repeated seizures, abnormal EEGs (electroencephalograms) and have a family history of seizures. In some forms of epilepsy the inherent capacity to inhibit seizures is genetically low, and the patient has spontaneous seizures. On the other hand, a patient who is under severe stress, neglecting health maintenance issues (proper diet and adequate sleep) may have seizures that are not epileptic in nature. The content of that individual's life creates enough stress to decrease the threshold for a seizure.

When content of life (stress) interacts with the brain and produces illness behavior, it can be difficult to pinpoint the behavioral determinant. Does the patient have a physiological illness, or is the content of life the major determinant of behavior? Can both be true? This type of situation highlights the significance of psychologists and psychiatrists working together to sort out specific determinants of behavior and to collaborate on the diagnosis/treatment of psychosomatic illnesses.

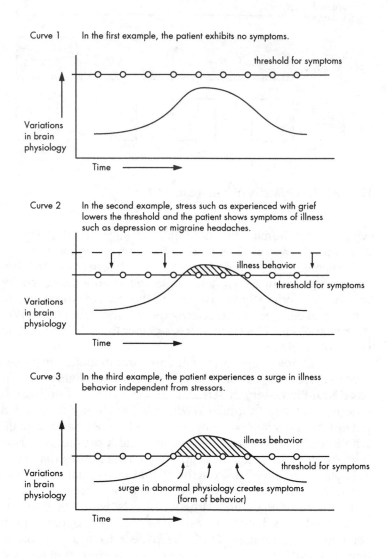

Curve 1   In the first example, the patient exhibits no symptoms.

threshold for symptoms

Variations in brain physiology

Time

Curve 2   In the second example, stress such as experienced with grief lowers the threshold and the patient shows symptoms of illness such as depression or migraine headaches.

illness behavior

threshold for symptoms

Variations in brain physiology

Time

Curve 3   In the third example, the patient experiences a surge in illness behavior independent from stressors.

illness behavior

threshold for symptoms

Variations in brain physiology

surge in abnormal physiology creates symptoms (form of behavior)

Time

Figure 5-2. Stress model.

The Open Model Algorithm

Groups of generators of behavior that determine basic human function are named, as follows, according to the type of behavior they govern.
Biological determinants govern:

- Self-mood and affectivity
- Instincts
- Cognitive behavior

Psychosocial determinants govern:

- Sense of belonging
- Sense of right and wrong

Spiritual determinants govern:

- Sense of what is important or meaningful

The three main areas of brain function—biological, psychosocial, and spiritual—have been mentioned earlier in this text. It is worth noting here that biological areas relate to all aspects of brain function:

1. All behavioral components in the brain are biological. The brain provides the biological form for psychological, social and spiritual behavior.
2. Because brain physiology dictates the form of behavior, any change in the form of behavior usually relates to biological determinants of behavior.
3. When there is a biological disruption in the brain, one or more independent generators of behavior in the brain will create behavior that may interrupt normal psychological, social or spiritual behaviors (i.e., the creation of a new form of behavior).[4]

In general, the content of an individual's life interacts with the psychological, social and spiritual generators of the brain. Life content can affect the **psychological aspect** of the brain in the following ways:

1. production of grief
2. posttraumatic stress disorder
3. shame
4. codependence
5. abusive relationships
6. memory—knowledge
7. total experience (Gestalt)
8. learning
9. beliefs (childhood or "core beliefs")
10. others

Life content can affect the **social aspect** of the brain in the following ways:

1. social isolation
2. guilt
3. legal degrees
4. social rejection
5. others

Life content can affect the **spiritual aspect** of the brain in the following ways:

1. lack of spiritual awareness or focus
2. spiritual isolation

Since the foundations for all behavior are biological, it makes sense to establish physiological stability before examining the content of one's life. Once the form of behavior is found to be stable, content of life can be examined to determine how it influences behavior.

It is reasonable to view the above behavior classifications as a hierarchy, with biological/genetic determinants providing the foundation for all behavior. Consideration of all three spheres of determinants comprises the open model of behavioral examination.

The open model can be summarized by the following algorithm:

1. Is the source biological? (based on the Medical Model?)
   - Yes . . . the source is linked with an independent generator of behavior, such as a major depressive cluster.
   - Refer to biological psychiatrist.
   - No . . . (go to next step)

2. Is unusual content of life (i.e., abuse, PTSD, high stress) present?
   - Yes . . . the major determinant may be stress over a variety of factors (i.e., divorce proceedings, death of a loved one), and stress decreases the threshold for all generators of behavior.
   - Refer to biological psychiatrist or therapist.
   - No . . . (go to next step)

3. Is a maladapative generator of behavior (i.e., codependence, social isolation) present?
   - Yes . . . the patient may have strong bonding generators of behavior that prevent him/her from leaving a "bad" relationship, resulting in demoralization and suicidal thoughts or "core beliefs" that result in a feeling of inferiority (i.e., "inferiority complex").
   - Refer to biological psychiatrist or therapist.
   - No . . . (go to next step)

4. Are spiritual problems present?
   - Yes . . . even individuals who feel well and have everything going their way may become suicidal if there is no "meaning" in their lives.
   - Refer to religious counselor.
   - No . . . reevaluate and return to Step 1.

Note in the open model algorithm that the hierarchical system is followed. First, biological determinants are queried (i.e., looking for generators of behavior that are independent of the personality matrix).[5] Second, psychosocial problems are investigated. Third, spiritual issues are examined.

Structural and Physiological Determinants

The basic structure and physiology of the brain determines behavior, with the human gene being the major determinant for human physiology. Genes have the capacity to think and make decisions in remarkable ways, and they direct the composition and form of every living creature. Like time-release capsules, genes are knit together in just the right sequence (i.e., the genetic timeline[6]) to uniquely shape individual growth and behavior.[7]

When egg and sperm come together (fertilization), life begins and the "genetic clock" is created. All biological instructions for a lifetime are encoded in a miraculous and instantaneous union. The winding of the genetic clock is performed by the maternal placenta, which provides the energy to fuel the genetic template.

Evidence for genetic determination of behavior is drawn from family history studies and DNA profiles. Such research allows early identification of at-risk individuals, encourages genetic counseling and provides clues about specific defects associated with particular illnesses.[8] For example, individuals who begin to experience recurrent bouts of asthma in their 20s might benefit from knowing about similar symptoms experienced by family members whose asthma attacks seemed to dissipate in their 40s and 50s.

Many neurological diseases are time-dependent. For instance, an individual with Huntington's chorea may be asymptomatic until age 45, when chorea-form (involuntary) movements and dementia develop, which can be fatal in only a few years. DNA analysis can show the presence of the Huntington's chorea gene. In fact, the future of illness behavior actually can be predicted by studying genes, because of the genetic timeline.

Several components can vary the effect of genetic or inherited determinants:

1. *Dominant and recessive traits*—These are hereditary patterns that relate to genetic penetrance (see no. 2). If there is only one gene of the recessive type, there is no clinical manifestation of a disorder. If there is one dominant gene, clinical manifestations are evident.

2. *Degree of genetic penetrance*—In some cases, variable penetrance is present, a genetic trait that falls somewhere between dominant effect (total expression) and recessive effect (absence of expression). Variable penetrance applies to dominant genes that do not always express themselves clinically.

3. *Amount of genetic loading*—This factor relates to the number of family members who manifest a particular trait. For instance, if every member of a patient's family has a genetic trait (i.e., bipolar disorder), there is 100 percent genetic loading, and there is 100 percent penetrance. If one parent has bipolar disorder, the offspring have a 20 percent chance of having this form of brain failure; if both parents have bipolar disorder, there is a 70 percent chance that the offspring will

bear the trait. In other words, the more often relatives share a trait, the more likely it is that offspring will carry the trait.

Other variables can have a powerful impact on genetic machinery:

- stress related to pregnancy or the birthing process
- head trauma
- illness during infancy (i.e., fever, seizure)
- space-occupying lesions in or near the brain (i.e., tumors, circulatory malformations, aneurysms, subdural hematomas)

Analysis of basic brain structures shows that behavior also is determined by the region of the brain in which it originates (see below). Primitive behavior emanates from the brain stem, with the higher functions initiating in the cortex and progressing to the frontal lobes where the awareness center receives inputs from many sources.

Brain stem	Regulates primitive behavior, such as respiration and heart rate
Midbrain	Controls robotics capabilities
Occipital lobes	Control visual inputs
Temporal/parietal lobes	Regulate sensory inputs, memory and language
Cortex/frontal lobes	Regulate executive function and awareness

The well known developmental psychologist, Jean Piaget, conducted extensive psychological testing to portray how the brain acquires increased capacities over time.[9] His findings revealed that parts of the brain develop at a particular rate and that the rate defines individual capacities for awareness/executive function, memory, language/cognitive skill and robotics.[10] Pediatricians use developmental tables to monitor rates of childhood growth and development.

Nonstructural Determinants

Once the basic structure of the brain has been determined (i.e., physiology of the neuron), nonstructural influences on behavior must be considered. Physical variables that alter brain biology predominantly affect the form of behavior; psychosocial variables alter brain psychology, and predominantly affect content of behavior.

Establishing specific determinants of behavior beyond the structure of the brain has been the source of great controversy in psychiatry since the early 1900s when Sigmund Freud first proposed his psychoanalytic theories. Theories with psychological or social bases have been advanced by many others.[11] From a scientific point of view, no psychodynamic or Freudian theory has ever been shown to be a valid source of illness behavior.

In order to illustrate how psychosocial theories can be interpreted into the biological model, let's look at stress (Fig. 5-2, page 80).[12] Basically, all stress reduces the threshold for illness. One nonstructural determinant of behavior may involve maladaptive behavior that results in high stress on the brain. Therefore, high stress can cause brain dysfunction in the presence of normal brain structure and chemistry. Because people have different vulnerable generators of behavior and differing levels of stress thresholds, however, stress affects everyone uniquely. It may manifest in countless ways, from depression, panic attacks, addictive behavior to psychosomatic problems.

It is important to note that the mixture of patients seen by therapists includes those with illness behavior and those with maladaptive behavior. It is essential that patients understand the nature of their particular illness so that all treatment options can be explored fully with the therapist. Because patients are consumers of health care, they must be prepared to understand their problem well enough to make choices that fit their unique needs.[13]

Patients who have a low genetic vulnerability for illness and a high profile for maladaptive behavior respond best to psychological therapies. In these cases the major determinants of behavior are not physiological (involving form), but psychological as a result of stress that affects content of life. Mild forms of most illness, especially in high-stress societies, usually respond to psychological therapies that provide the following:

1. stress reduction
2. psychological support
3. assistance in developing realistic life strategies
4. help in changing maladaptive forms of behavior, such as codependence
5. countering of unrealistic expectations

Psychosocial disorders that affect brain function are similar to psychosomatic disorders; for both types of disorders the main determinant of dysfunction is stress.

Stress reduces the threshold for illness that intersects with the physiology of illness. In the case of psychosocial disorders, reduction of the threshold might produce depression. In the case of psychosomatic disorders, reduction of the threshold might produce migraine headaches, for which biofeedback may be appropriate. For spontaneously occurring migraines, where physiology is the major determinant, medical treatment is appropriate. For patients who have features of both stress and physiological determinants, combined therapies may be utilized (i.e., psychological and medical treatment).

In the case of psychosomatic disorders (disorders that stem from psycho [mind] and somatic [body] interactions) and psychosocial disorders, real *physiology* of the body and mind is involved. These are not "functional" disorders that are "imagined" by either patients or physicians.

Examples of psychosomatic disorders include asthma, migraine headaches, irritable bowel syndrome, and low back pain. Note that all these disorders share at least one feature—a spasm reflex, which often is induced by stress. Asthma is typified by bronchial spasms; migraine headaches, by arterial spasms; irritable bowel syndrome, by large bowel spasms; low back pain, by muscle spasms.

The same neuropsychiatric principles that apply to general psychiatry also apply to psychosomatic medicine.

In Curve 1 of Fig. 5-2, the illness is in a latent or quiescent phase. In Curve 2, the primary determinant is the physiology of illness, resulting in spontaneous migraines, asthma attacks, irritable bowel syndrome, or low back pain.

Some patients' illnesses reflect only Curve 3 and, therefore, are not psychosomatic. Other patients, whose illnesses include only Curve 2, have disorders that are purely psychosomatic. Most patients, however, include contributions from both Curve 2 and Curve 3, depending on the phase of their illness. Obviously, treatment focus depends on determinants of illness.

Biological determinants beyond the genetic foundation are physical elements that influence the form of behavior, or promote independent generators that interfere with normal behavior. In other words, the capacity for illness is genetically determined (unless it occurs secondary to medical illness), but there are biological variables that influence the genetic expression of illness.

Following is a list of the biological determinants that exist outside the genetic foundation:

1. Cyclical variables related to behavioral illness (genetic)
2. Cyclical variables that influence illness behavior
3. Psychological stressors
4. Hormonal and vitamin fluctuations
5. Systemic illness (including substance abuse)

Cyclical variables (related to behavioral illness): The cycling of illness can push the physiology of the brain above its threshold for illness. Certain psychiatric illnesses, especially panic/anxiety disorders and mood disorders, tend to cycle or follow predictable patterns. Cycling may occur as often as every 48 hours or as infrequently as every 5 to 10 years or longer. This type of cycling is genetically determined or internally regulated.

Cyclical variables (that influence illness behavior): These include:

1. **advancing age**, which generally causes patients to cycle into more vulnerable states for illness
2. **illnesses that are cyclical** (i.e., allergies), which put patients into physiological stress and increase vulnerability to brain dysfunction
3. **sensitivity to different times of day** (diurnal changes), which may affect an individual's emotional outlook and ability to function according to the particular time of day. Some people are depressed and lethargic in the morning but experience a "recharge" later in the day; others are "rarin' to go" in the early morning but run out of steam toward late afternoon.
4. **environmental temperature extremes** (i.e., severe heat during Arizona summers), which affect brain function
5. **dramatic barometric changes**, which can cause arthritis-related inflammation and pain that affect brain function

Circadian stressors: These include the two major cyclical variables that influence illness behavior.

1. **The sleep-wake cycle** (circadian rhythm) is an important function of normal brain activity, but any disturbance in this pattern can provide stress and decrease the threshold for illness. Whenever individuals are sleep-deprived, they will experience heightened levels of tension, anxiety, over-

reactivity and obsessiveness. Numerous elements can disrupt circadian rhythms:

- Sleep disorders
- Self-imposed sleep deprivation
- Seasonal weather changes
- Jet lag
- Physiologic stress, such as medical illness
- Psychological stress (severe)
- Vocational shift changes

2. **Seasonal weather changes** have an especially significant impact on behavior. Seasonal affective disorder (SAD) is a mood disorder that occurs in response to varying lengths of day.

There probably is a connection between seasonal variables and circadian variables. The variable that occurs during seasonal changes, which disrupts circadian rhythm, is the varying length of day. The sleep-wake cycle is dependent on cyclical releases of increased melatonin at night and increased cortisol during the day. During the month of October, however, there is an acceleration in shortening of the day, and in May there is an acceleration in the lengthening of the day.[14] The rapid change in length of day has a destabilizing effect on normal brain functioning. When the length of day changes, the sleep-wake cycle must adjust to different patterns of melatonin release and other variables. This adjustment phase stresses the brain and probably is the cause of SAD. (Not surprisingly, May and October have the highest suicide rates, compared to other months of the year.)[15]

As latitude increases, so does the incidence of SAD. This can be an anticipated phenomenon since the higher the latitude, the more extreme are the changes in length of day. For example, in the higher latitudes of Alaska, near Barrow's Point, it is dark all day in the deepest part of winter and light all night in mid-summer.[16]

Treatment for SAD is simple—trick the brain into thinking the days are longer in winter and shorter in summer. In the winter, bright lights can be used in the morning to lengthen the day. In the summer, the bedroom can be darkened to lengthen the night. As mentioned earlier, other weather-induced physical stressors are excessive summer heat and barometric changes that affect inflammatory illness, such as rheumatoid arthritis.

Psychological stressors: As described earlier, these are manifested in maladaptive behavior, such as poor coping skills or strategies with life, grief reaction, posttraumatic stress disorder, or abuse. In addition to reducing the threshold for psychiatric disorders, stress can decrease the threshold for all types of illnesses and can produce a cascade affect for illness (i.e., tension or migraine headaches caused by stress). When the major determinant for illness is stress, the illness is designated as psychosomatic, as previously described.

Hormonal and vitamin fluctuations: It is well known that hormone imbalances and vitamin deficiencies provide physiological stress to the brain. For women, generators of the brain that are sensitive to stress may manifest neuropsychiatric symptoms, most notably during instances of rapid hormonal shifts—menarche, pre-menstrually, following childbirth, and at menopause.

Low thyroid level (hypothyroidism) is another form of hormonal imbalance, which can cause symptoms of depression identical to those seen in cases of primary or genetic depression. (Remember, when the brain fails in its usual capacities, clinical presentation is the same, regardless of cause.)

The effects of vitamin deficiency can be exemplified by inadequate supplies of vitamin B1 (thiamine). Thiamine deficiency is particularly common in alcoholism and associated brain dysfunctions, including Wernicke's encephalopathy and Korsakoff's psychosis. Wernicke's encephalopathy results in confusion, agitation, double vision and difficulty with gait. Korsakoff's psychosis causes amnesia (memory loss) and confabulation (fabrication of information).

Systemic illness: Because the primary function of all organ systems is to support brain function, systemic illnesses always provide a stress on the brain. In fact, 10 to 15 percent of individuals who present to their physicians with medical problems have neuropsychiatric symptoms.[17] As age decreases brain reserve, the impact of systemic illness increases. For example, a urinary tract infection in a young woman may cause irritability whereas the same illness in an elderly woman may cause psychosis.

Congestive heart failure (CHF) is an example of systemic illness that affects the brain. This condition renders the heart incapable of supplying the body with adequate oxygen for body tissues; the most direct result is decreased oxygen delivery to the brain. Patients experience shortness of breath and fluid retention, which frequently are accompanied by anxiety and depression.

Some medical illnesses, such as allergies or asthma, are cyclical. The physiological stress of an asthma attack, for example, can precipitate a panic attack, while the systemic stress of allergies can precipitate depression. In fact, some "alternative therapies" purport that allergic desensitization has antidepressant or antipsychotic effects.

Dependence on and/or overuse of alcohol, illegal drugs and prescribed medications can have a range of effects on brain function, depending on the type of substance being used. Agents such as alcohol, marijuana, cocaine, and heroin typically cause distorted states of euphoria, serenity, anxiety or panic; chronic use can lead to behavior resembling schizophrenia.[18]

Abuse of medically prescribed sedatives, such as Valium and Xanax, can result in depression, dizziness, confusion, stupor and coma.

Overuse of stimulants, such as Benzedrine and Ritalin, may cause increased blood pressure, irregular heart rate, tremors, hallucinations, and even circulatory collapse and death.[19]

Psychological/Social Determinants

The impacts of psychological and social determinants on behavior are numerous. As noted previously, psychological and social determinants relate to the content of life. From a psychological point of view, the content of life relates to the self (awareness) and interpersonal relationships. From a social point of view, some determinants relate to mores and the social mileu. Different regions of the brain create the form for the psychological and social content of life.

The Brain as an Organized System

To review, a generator of behavior is a group of brain cells that works together for a common function, such as memory function, language function, and mood function. Individual personality is comprised of all superimposed generators as they form the matrix of behavior. Personality is comprised of both the overt behavior that others can see and aspects that can be only personally perceived (i.e., the totality of all generators of behavior in the brain).

The basic building block of behavior, the brain cell, and the structure of the brain are the components that define the self, interpersonal/psychosocial relationships and spiritual awareness.

From a systems point of view (when many generators of behavior act together), awareness and control of executive function are the overriding determinants of human behavior. As stated in Chapter 4, awareness is a sustained reflective thought. The executive function aspect of awareness (the capacity to direct and control brain function) has directive capacities. For instance, when a therapist asks a patient, "How do you feel?" the therapist is asking the executive function to focus on emotional inputs related to the self. In the Mental Status Exam, emotional reactivity is described as "affect."[20]

Therapists can help patients improve their psychological outlook by identifying negative thoughts in the awareness center.[21] Cognitive therapy helps patients to replace negative thoughts with positive thoughts (i.e., affirmations), to distract awareness with positive thoughts or to focus on goal-oriented tasks.[22]

Awareness also is influenced by emotional coloring (intensity of a given thought), provided by the amygdala, the group of neurons in the temporal lobe that adds emotional dimension to cognitive thought. Emotions registered in response to certain inputs to the awareness center relate to an appropriate range of intensity of thought. Instincts influence emotional coloring.

For instance, if a husband sees his wife with another man, the corresponding rage or jealousy is an instinct designed to preserve an interpersonal bond for reproductive purposes. Or, the desire to work and accumulate material wealth corresponds to the survival instinct. The relevance of the brain and its effect on evolution is another facet of awareness. Although the brain is isolated from the outside world, it has evolved to reflect external reality and, as mentioned in Chapter 4, provides a subjective assignment to all external and internal sensory inputs.[23]

The more we learn about the brain and the nature of existence, the more difficult it is to define "reality." In a sense, all awareness and all reality is virtual, and virtual reality generated by computers is bound to emulate human reality someday.

Evolution of the Content of Life

Although genetic determinants dictate approximately 80 percent of human behavior, the content of life has a major impact on behavior as well. It is not always obvious how powerfully social forces mold individual behavior. When assessing behavioral problems, however, in addition to considering biological influences, it is just as important to ensure balance between self-generated needs and social factors.

For example, medical treatment of schizophrenia is limited, leading to the diagnosis of "chronic mental illness." Schizophrenics tend to be socially isolated and lacking in interpersonal skills. Social support systems have been shown to be very effective in helping patients deal with schizophrenia. Networks of support groups, peers, social workers, and therapists can prevent relapse and hospitalization.

If biology of the brain is stable (meaning, there are no independent generators of behavior interfering with the personality structure), the search for stressors that might cause an imbalance between the personal and social needs is initiated during standard psychiatric assessments. (See the open model algorithm on page 81.)

Psychological problems related to the self can involve self-esteem, codependence, life strategies and the capacity to cope with stress. (See "Basic Strategies of Life" on page 94.) The traditional psychodynamic approach investigates psychological processes (i.e., denial, projection, and rationalization) as contributors to disorders of the self.

The biological approach does not exclude psychodynamic ideas but includes them in the open model. The following study of codependence illustrates the "open brain" model where the impact of psychological *and* biological factors on brain function is considered. When psychological processes provide the source of stress or maladaptive behavior, psychological therapies (i.e., biofeedback, psychotherapy, and group therapy) are appropriate.

Codependence is defined as an individual's focus on another individual's priorities, lack of healthy personal boundaries, and decreased capacity to communicate needs. The following generators of behavior, when taken to extremes, can result in codependence:

1. *Instinctive generators*, exemplified by the maternal instinct that gives top priority to children's needs at the expense of the mother's needs.
2. *Illness generators*, exemplified by depression, exhibited by individuals who feel they must comply with the demands of others, regardless of their own desires. Guilt behavior generated by depression makes patients easily manipulated to conform to the desires of others.

Basic Strategies of Life

The Biological Psychiatry Institute recommends the following 10 health maintenance concepts as basic strategies to maximize the quality of life:

1. Read *Brain Basics: An Integrated Biological Approach to Understanding and Assessing Human Behavior.*

Brain Basics offers strategies in coping and dealing with human behavior as well as providing a basis for understanding and assessing behavior. It also expresses the concept that there is no perfect brain and that it is normal for everyone to experience brain failure at some point in life.

In terms of assessing behavior, consideration of the impact of form and content is relevant. If a behavioral problem is biologically determined, then focus on the form of behavior follows. If a behavioral problem is psychologically determined, then focus on the content of life follows. If a psychological focus is used to treat a biologically determined disorder, however, frustration and failure will follow.

Likewise, if you regularly deal with an individual who has active behavioral illness, you are bound to experience frustration and bewilderment. Individuals with behavioral illness do not have executive control over their behavior (they cannot control their behavior through their own will). When you address illness behavior, you quickly discover that rational thought is absent.

There is no rational way to deal directly with irrational or illness behavior. Supportive but minimal involvement is usually best. Since illness behavior frequently is outside the individual's scope of awareness, referral for help is difficult, but the focus of treatment should be biologically based.

2. Maintain balance among the three major determinants of behavior—biological, psychosocial, and spiritual.
3. Maintain cyclical instinctual generators through healthy diet and adequate rest.
4. Exercise (aerobic and musculoskeletal) four times a week.

In our society aerobic activity is emphasized for good reason, but musculoskeletal relationships must not be overlooked. Muscle tone and posture are important for health, too, and are the basis for chiropractic medicine. (I frequently send patients either to a physical therapist or chiropractor for physical therapy.)

The brain is designed to maintain body systems in specific balance, and when the body is "out of whack" (a phenomenon I often see in my practice), muscle spasms with associated pain and tension can result because the brain is "frustrated" in its instinctual attempts to maintain anatomical balance. In order to maintain this balance, I recommend the following types of exercise be practiced at least four times a week.

   a. Aerobic exercise to strengthen "inside" (cardiovascular) muscles (20 minutes per day)
   b. Muscle toning exercises to strengthen "outside" (musculoskeletal) muscles (20 minutes per day)

Basic Strategies of Life continued

Exercise has been shown to enhance health and mood. Aerobic exercise, four times per week for 20 to 30 minutes, will utilize 80 to 90 percent of cardiovascular capacity. Walking at a brisk pace is an easy, inexpensive form of aerobic exercise, but any exercise is beneficial. The most important aspect of exercising is getting into the habit of doing it. If you do not enjoy exercise, you probably will not pursue any form of it, no matter how motivated you may be. So, try different kinds of activities until you find something you enjoy.

5. Minimize financial stress by maintaining low debt level and minimal expenses.
6. Avoid alcohol and intoxicating drugs.
7. Understand the dominant generators of behavior in your brain (i.e., personality characteristics).
8. Utilize your executive function (ability to change your focus of awareness) to maximize positive thoughts and minimize negative thoughts. Meditation and/or prayer can be helpful in this regard.
9. Maintain a balanced intake of vitamins, minerals, proteins, and carbohydrates through diet and/or dietary supplements.
10. Maintain a continuing focus on spiritual thoughts and values through education (get plenty of exercise for your brain).

Education is the spiritual component that enhances the process of learning, understanding, and communicating throughout our entire lives. This process can occur in a formal classroom setting or through reading, games, lively discussion, and countless other ways. Make the most of the miraculous mechanism that allows each of us to share the awareness (sustained reflective thought) within ourselves with other individuals, reflecting existence through subjective impressions.

---

3. *Social generators*, exemplified by an almost overwhelming (and crippling) sense of obligation to certain individuals.
4. *Awareness generators*, exemplified by an individual who ignores incoming signals from the awareness center and denies all personal needs.
5. *"Core belief" generators*, exemplified by low self-esteem and negative beliefs about the self and caused by traumatic childhood experiences. Childhood beliefs influence personality behavior in that automatic thoughts may occur that are based on a "core belief." Automatic thoughts that someone is "no good" can result in a codependent condition, i.e., an individual does not deserve to determine his or her own priorities.

Spiritual Determinants

Evolutionary theory states that humankind evolved from the animal kingdom as a social species with the special capacity of awareness, which gives individuals the ability to appreciate life or existence. When humankind progressed from an environment of sheer survival in the animal kingdom to the human kingdom, spirituality evolved—the quest for inner peace and relationships of depth and relevance with other individuals. (One of the greatest spiritual leaders of all time, Jesus Christ, taught the basic principles of spiritual humanism.) When an individual discards spiritual elements of life, animalistic instincts dominate, paving the way for war and inhumanity. When spiritual ideals are pursued and upheld, goodness results.

Many determinants affect an individual's spiritual outlook:

1. Perception of the meaning of life
2. Importance of relationships with others
3. Appreciation of life itself
4. Experience of oneness or connection with humankind or the universe, in general
5. Experience of the joy of life; the capacity to celebrate life
6. Internalization of the goodness and dignity inherent in all individuals
7. Capacity to accept life circumstances
8. Belief in a superior being (i.e., God) and/or respect for the miracle of life that satisfies an individual's spiritual needs

An individual who presents with complaints of dissatisfaction with life and a feeling of emptiness usually is trying to cope with multiple spiritual stressors. When such factors are present, prescribed "therapy" focuses primarily on involvement with formalized religion or other sources designed to provide spiritual fulfillment.

Applying Determinants of Behavior

When individuals come to the Biological Psychiatry Institute exhibiting active psychiatric symptoms (behavior that reflects illness), all possible major determinants of the behavior are evaluated. This is done, using the following protocol (or algorithm):

1. Determination of relationship between symptoms
2. Assessment of psychosocial/spiritual balance; that is, analysis of major losses, social isolation, high stressors
3. Evaluation of medical illnesses that may contribute to relapse
4. Evaluation of biological determinants, including:

   • intrinsic cycling
   • seasonal affects
   • adequacy of medication
   • potential side-effects of medications, such as low thyroid states produced as a side-effect of lithium

5. Development of treatment strategies, such as bright light therapy for winter (seasonal) depression; initiation of group therapy to deal with high stressors; referral to internist for evaluation for other illnesses

The two following examples illustrate how identification of determinants of behavior—through application of the open model—can lead to diagnosis and treatment of specific forms of brain failure.

Substance abuse/addiction[24]

"Substance abuse" is defined as maladaptive use of any substance that has an effect on behavior. "Addiction" is defined as the formation of an independent generator of behavior that creates the desire for a substance not normally required for survival. Both substance abuse and addiction are multifactoral problems in that they have many determinants of behavior. Fig. 5-3 (page 99) illustrates the elements that are determinants of substance abuse.

Most readers are familiar with the maladaptive use of drugs and alcohol, but let us look briefly at the adaptive use of these substances as a determinant of behavior. Studies of drug use by military men and women during the Vietnam War indicate that drugs, such as marijuana, may have helped prevent or minimize Posttraumatic Stress Disorder (PTSD). Understandably, these studies were unpopular with military leaders. It was purported that drugs modified the emotional reactivity that caused PTSD.

In some medical circles moderate use of alcohol is believed to enhance social functioning and even prolong life. Manic patients who need sleep may use alcohol for its sedative effects. Maladaptive use of alcohol, however, can precipitate aggressive behavior, increased depression, auto accidents, and toxic effects on the nervous system, liver, gastrointestinal tract, and pancreas.

It is not uncommon for individuals to begin drinking on a social basis. After they discover the calming effects of alcohol, they may begin to use it to treat depression, insomnia or anxiety. There actually may be stages of determinants leading to addiction.

Addiction always is maladaptive, meaning that—apart from personality—the nucleus accumbens produces the desire to use a substance that is *not* ordinarily desired for normal physiological functioning. The likelihood of substance addiction involves genetics, amount of substance used and time of its use, as well as social environment.

Suicide

The consideration of ending one's own life reflects an adaptable capacity of the brain to cope with stress or pain. All individuals experience mild forms of instinctively generated suicidal thoughts. When suicidal thoughts become severe, multiple sources and determinants of behavior must be examined. If suicidal behavior is caused by illness,[25] then the illness is treated and other determinants, such as social and interpersonal stress, are evaluated simultaneously. If the suicidal behavior manifests in response to overwhelming stress, patients can be referred for counseling.[26] Acute stress reaction can alter an individual's perceptions of the future, capacity to cope with stress, feelings of being empowered and capacity to experience pleasure. Most completed suicides are secondary to behavior that is illness-related, combined with other determinants, such as substance abuse.

The capacity to be suicidal (a generator located in the temporal lobes of the brain) is an instinct that usually is dormant in most individuals.[27] It has been shown that there are familial tendencies toward a vulnerability to be suicidal, meaning that there are genes that actually decrease the threshold for suicide. Various mechanisms can decrease the threshold so that suicidal thoughts become manifest, or an individual becomes aware of suicidal thoughts. These mechanisms include:

1. Psychological and/or physiological stress (drugs, pain, etc.)
2. Major depression

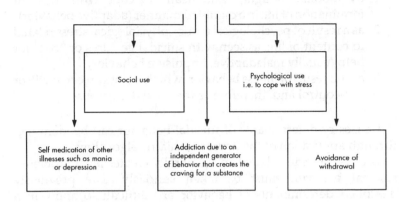

Figure 5-3. Causes of substance use.

3. Obsessive-compulsive disorder
4. Self-induced factors (malingering seen with sociopaths)[28]
5. Psychosis

Those who consider suicide for relief of psychological and/or physiological stress typically use alcohol maladaptively, have experienced divorce, severe financial loss, or prolonged social isolation. When psychological stressors are a major determinant in suicidal behavior, psychotherapy is indicated and normally addresses the following issues:

1. Coping skills
2. Supportive functions
3. Strategies of life
4. Codependence
5. Development of social support systems
6. "Core beliefs" leading to maladaptive automatic thoughts

When drug abuse is a major determinant, drug rehabilitation and Alcoholics Anonymous are recommended. When chronic illness (such as cancer) causes suicidal behavior, group therapy is recommended. When a brain disorder is the major cause of suicidal behavior, medical treatment is recommended. Supportive care and spiritual focus also are important.

In short, the brain has the capacity to produce suicidal thoughts. There are three main ways suicidal thoughts can be activated:

1. by rational thought, as a means to cope with stress or termination of life in a dignified manner (adaptive behavior)
2. as a result of psychological and/or physiological stress related to content of life, as seen with suicidal gestures or "cries for help (usually maladaptive, impulsive behavior)
3. as the result of illness behavior, which is not subject to will or self-control and, therefore, is the most dangerous

Causes or determinants of suicidal behavior can be identified through application of the neuropsychiatric algorithms.

Because suicide is lethal and generally creates legal problems, suicidal behavior must be taken seriously. The previously described determinants of behavior are difficult to apply in a practical sense. An individual simply may be manipulative or sending up a "call for help," but this never can be assumed. Extreme caution always is necessary in dealing with suicidal patients.

Summary

The open model for determinants of behavior examines all possible effects on behavior. These can be categorized as biological determinants (relating to form) or psychosocial/spiritual determinants (relating to content of life).

The foundation of behavior is genetic, which determines the basic structure and biochemical organization of the brain, as well as the genetic timeline. Beyond this foundation are physical elements, which affect the biology of the brain or forms of behavior, including:

1. Cyclical variables
2. Circadian stressors
3. Psychological stressors
4. Hormonal and vitamin fluctuations
5. Systemic illness (including substance abuse)

Examples of application of the open model are provided relative to substance abuse and suicide.

References

1. A gestalt experience is a total experience, more than just the summation of separate parts of individual experience. For example, eating dinner in Venice, Italy is a unique gestalt experience that amounts to more than the place, people, language, aroma or taste of the food.
2. Generally, the clinical signs of brain failure are the same, regardless of the cause of brain failure. For example, the symptoms of major depression secondary to a stroke are the same as major depression secondary to a bipolar mood disorder.
3. *Diagnostic and statistical manual of mental disorders.* 4th edition. Washington, DC: The American Psychiatric Association; 1994:327.
4. Major depression is an example of an independent generator that interrupts normal function. Psychologically, major depression causes low self-esteem. Socially, it causes social isolation. Spiritually, it causes loss of spiritual "connectedness."
5. The personality "matrix" is a composite of behavior comprised of separate generators of behavior.
6. The genetic timeline influences basic human functioning. During the early years of life, there is a tendency to focus on biological function (i.e., reproduction). During the middle years of life, emphasis usually is placed on social/industrial functions. In later years more attention is given to spiritual function. For every individual there is an overlap among these three areas. Psychologists or social scientists refer to the transitions from one functional stage to the next as "passages of life."
7. Some biologists theorize that the aggressiveness of humankind that leads to wars is imparted by genes as a means of population control, according to the same pattern seen in the animal kingdom.
8. Michels R, Marzuk PM. Progress in psychiatry. *The New England Journal of Medicine* 1993;552–560.
9. Pediatricians use developmental charts based on Piaget's work to plot expected neurological development of infants and children.
10. In medical school every physician is taught to use an infant/child developmental milestone table. As development of the nervous system follows the genetic timeline, nervous system function predictably advances. This table can be reviewed in "Mental retardation: an introduction" by Francis Pirozzolo (In: Vinken PJ, Bruyn GW, Klawans HL, eds. *Handbook of clinical neurology.* Amsterdam: Elsevier Science Publishers, 1985:7).
11. *Introduction to Psychology* by Clifford Morgan and Richard King (New York: McGraw-Hill Book Company, 1975), 465–471, describes Carl Jung's analytic theory, Alfred Adler's psychological theory, Karen Horney's basic anxiety theory, and self theories by Maslow and Rogers.

12. Stress is a challenging force on the brain that tends to disrupt the brain's structure or biochemistry.

13. Generally, individuals seek psychiatric help to control illness or prevent suffering. An individual with a behavioral problem in combination with normal brain function probably would not consult a biological psychiatrist. Similarly, an individual with normal cardiopulmonary function would not seek advice from a cardiologist about training for a marathon.

14. Light suppresses melatonin, which can (in extreme cases) lead to hyperactivity. Darkness facilitates the release of melatonin, which can trigger depression.

15. SAD also is played out in the animal kingdom. For example, in the winter bears become lethargic, irritable, somnolent, have increased appetite, and eventually go into hibernation (symptoms and activities equivalent to human depression). When the days lengthen in the summer, bears become hypersexual and have increased appetite (symptoms and activities equivalent to human hyperactivity).

16. It also is worth noting that some researchers feel that lunar cycles can lead to psychiatric disorders, especially the monthly occurrence of the full moon. (The term, "lunatic," is derived from the Latin word, "luna," which means "moon.") Although scientific studies do not confirm any "full moon syndrome," psychiatrists and emergency room specialists are conditioned (through experience) to expect an increase in patients with psychiatric symptoms when the full moon appears.

17. When the term "neuropsychiatric" is used in medical literature, it usually refers to one of three definitions of brain dysfunction: (a) clusters (i.e., depression), (b) traditional psychosis, or (c) cognitive dysfunction.

18. Freedman AM, Kaplan HI, Sadock BJ. Organic brain syndromes. In: *Modern Synopsis of Comprehensive Textbook of Psychiatry II.* 2nd ed. Baltimore: The Williams & Wilkins Co; 1977:559.

19. Freedman, Kaplan, Sadock: 558–559.

20. Emotional affectivity, which can be described as sad, happy, angry, anxious, and many other terms, is the normal emotional response to emotional input to the brain. Examples include:

    - "I'm angry at my husband."
    - "I'm anxious about paying income tax."
    - "I'm happy about a vacation trip to Paris."

21. Frequently, emphasis on therapy for biologically based problems can worsen psychosocial problems. Biological therapy typically is designed to maximize treatment response and minimize side effects, whereas psychosocial therapy seeks to reduce stress, decrease maladaptive behaviors, and develop new life strategies.

    For example, an individual with demoralization syndrome may work on positive affirmations, but the resultant positive outlook may aggravate anticipatory anxiety of failure. After patients learn how to monitor determinants within their control (i.e., biological and psychosocial), it is wise to focus on spiritual determinants, which can provide ways to cope with factors outside human control.

22. Books, such as *The Power of Positive Thinking* by Norman Vincent Peale and *The Language of Letting Go* by Melody Beattie, can help individuals utilize executive function to discard negative thoughts that impair healthy functioning.

23. Subjective assignments also can be elicited purely on the basis of thought or experience, without any external input. This was proven in the 1930s when electrodes were applied to the temporal lobes of patients in an awake state. These patients heard sounds, voices, and underwent religious experiences without any external input.

24. Substance abuse and addiction provide an intriguing application to the open model of determinants of behavior. Addiction is possibly the most misunderstood disorder in psychiatry. "Just say no" exemplifies our culture's ignorance about addiction, which is a medical disorder that is *not* subject to will or self-control.

25. All illness produced by demoralization syndrome, such as panic disorder, can decrease the threshold for suicide.

26. Stress may generate many brain reactions, including anxiety, fear, panic attacks, suicidal thoughts, or any generator of behavior that is sensitive to stress.

27. The following factors can influence suicidal thoughts in a negative manner:

    - Hopelessness and anxiety
    - Social isolation
    - Substance abuse
    - Age (especially adolescence and postretirement)
    - Race (especially Caucasian)
    - Gender (especially male)

28. The DSM-IV (page 683) says that "the essential feature of malingering is the *intentional* production of false . . . physical or psychological symptoms motivated by external incentives . . . ".

6
Major Brain Disorders, Part I

Canst thou not minister to a mind diseased,
Pluck from the memory a rooted sorrow,
Raze out the written troubles of the brain,
And with some sweet oblivious antidote
Cleanse the stuffed bosom of that perilous stuff
Which weighs upon the heart?

William Shakespeare
Macbeth

The target of medical therapies is to control independent generators of behavior ("mind-diseased") that interfere with normal personality behavior ("heart").

Robert A. Williams, M.D.

Major brain disorders, or illnesses,[1] include those classifications of abnormality that are most common and have the potential to cause severe symptoms or suicide.[2] Primary causes of brain disorders are genetic. Secondary causes of behavioral illness are trauma, infection, multiple sclerosis, Alzheimer's disease, stroke, cerebral aneurysms, arteriovenous malformations, and many others.

In order to be defined as an "illness," the disorder must be chronic (with at least one or two documented episodes) and occur separate from life circumstance and personality.[3] For example, if an individual with a presumed low threshold for depression is depressed because of severe stress and grief over the death of a loved one, the individual is not considered "ill." Rather, a normal psychological grieving process is underway and prescribed treatment would include supportive psychotherapy and spiritual counseling.[4]

Many medical professionals refer to "functional" brain disorders as those that are caused by psychological mechanisms, as opposed to "organic" disorders that are caused by identifiable physical mechanisms. Neuropsychiatrists[5] never refer to brain disorders as being either functional or organic, because everything produced by the brain has an organic foundation and can be evaluated according to the Williams Brain Model. (See "Functional vs. Organic Brain Failure" on page 107 for further discussion about this issue.)

Major brain disorders are *neurologically based*. While there is nothing unique about the scientific concept of illness affecting the brain, there are several very specific ways in which psychosocial forces not only influence but exacerbate negative attitudes toward brain failure:

1. The **social stigma** of being "mentally ill" generally is made worse by the media and has a negative impact on societal attitudes, employment opportunities, and coverage by/compensation from insurance companies.
2. The foundational elements guiding **psychiatric training programs** in the United States are obsolete. They must be restructured to emphasize treatment of brain disorders by a new specialty that combines neurology and psychiatry under the auspices of internal medicine. Currently, internists, neurologists, and family physicians are not trained to treat most brain disorders.
3. Our nation's **constitutional laws** prevent the imposition of treatment for brain disorders except in narrowly defined situations that typically follow formal commitment proceedings.

Major brain disorders commonly are viewed as primarily influencing emotional well-being or interpersonal relationships. More accurately, a disease process that affects the brain includes components that impact both emotional *and* physical health.[6] For example, major depressive disorders cause irritable mood and emotional overreactivity to others; advanced depression also can affect motor activity and sometimes result in a catatonic state. A neurological disorder, such as Parkinson's disease, initially may affect motor function (characterized by tremors, slowed movement, muscle rigidity, and gait instability) and affect emotions only in the later stages of illness as the disease cuts across more generators of behavior.

A number of elements define specific major brain disorders:

- Clusters of signs and symptoms
- Age of onset of illness[7]
- Course of illness
- Response to medication

Functional vs. Organic Brain Failure

All internal brain activity and externally expressed activity is founded on *organic function*, since the brain is an organic body. The classification known as "functional" brain failure, indicating psychological dysfunction, has no scientific basis. The label, "functional brain failure," may serve merely as a sophisticated way for medical professionals to transfer treatment responsibility when they cannot determine any "organic" cause of patient symptoms. Even so, a neurologist may examine a catatonic patient and document the following in his office notes: "No localizing findings. MRI of the brain is normal. All physical findings, vital signs, and lab work are normal. Refer patient to psychiatrist, as findings suggest functional cause of behavior."

Another diagnostic note commonly found in a neurologist's office documentation would be "deficit does not fit known neuroanatomical pattern." This might be accompanied by the conclusion that the patient's disorder is "functional." It is important to point out that the majority of neuropsychiatric disorders can cause a broad array of symptoms that do *not* fit traditional neuroanatomic patterns. For instance, a patient with anorexia nervosa will "see" her body as overweight even though her visual mechanisms are intact. Or, a patient with conversion blindness who cannot "see" will have visual reflexes that are intact. (Forty percent of patients with conversion reaction who are diagnosed as "functional" are later found to have multiple sclerosis or another type of neurological disorder.) Although neither anorexia nervosa or conversion blindness conforms to neuroanatomic patterns, it is inappropriate to classify these disorders as functional.

- Results of physiologic testing (i.e., sleep studies)
- Family history[8]

There are 10 brain disorders for which we at the Biological Psychiatry Institute and others in neuropsychiatric settings are most frequently consulted. Chapter 6 provides a description of the five disorders that are most commonly associated with biological psychiatry:

1. Mood disorders
2. Anxiety disorders
3. Obsessive Compulsive Disorder
4. Schizophrenia
5. Attention Deficit Disorder

Chapter 7 provides a description of five common brain disorders that are not usually associated with biological psychiatry:

1. Personality disorders
2. Sleep disorders
3. Delirium
4. Dementia
5. Structural deficits, addiction, and permanent metabolic deficits

A special section in Chapter 7 addresses childhood brain disorders.

Mood Disorders

Summary: Mood disorders occur when the limbic system is underactivated (causing depression) or overactivated (causing mania) or both (causing a mixed state).

The basic brain cell mechanisms in the limbic system that cause mood swings are not well understood.[9] One theory proposes that cells causing depression are "down-regulated", or have too few receptors (resulting in a slow firing rate of brain cells).[10] Cells that cause mania have too many receptors (resulting in a fast firing rate. As the cycles of mania increase and the firing rate of brain cells picks up speed, there may be a continued enhancing effect called "kindling."[11] Kindling is believed to lead to rapid cycling similar to the process that occurs with seizure disorders.

The onset of a mood disorder may not be obvious, because there is overlap between normal mood and a mild form of mood disorder. The brain also has a normal fluctuation of mood or activity level, as reflected in "good days" or "bad days" that all of us experience.

Mood disorders are disorders of brain activation. Within this classification of brain disorder there is a wide range of clinical syndromes, from "psychotic depression with delirium" to "mania with psychosis." Generally, however, the three primary classifications of mood disorders—depression, mania, and mixed states—will be discussed here.

Typically, depressed patients experience low energy, slowed thinking, decreased ability to concentrate, and low self-esteem.[12] This state causes a total loss of appreciation of anything that might create pleasure.[13] Patients in a manic state experience high energy, sharpened thinking, increased ability to concentrate and high self-esteem.[14] Those who have a mixed (manic-depressive) mood state exhibit symptoms of both depression and mania, which may present as an activated depression or even as a psychosis.[15]

Mood disorders are cyclical in that they do not typically continue without interruption. Most patients usually are symptom-free between illness cycles, while others experience chronic residual depression. Behavior during an illness cycle changes so dramatically that the patient may appear to experience a different personality. The cycling quality can be a source of confusion, especially for family members, loved ones, and patients themselves. Following are several examples of the types of misunderstandings that cycling moods can cause:

- **Marital instability** During courtship an individual may appear easy-going and agreeable. After marriage, however, the same individual may become tense, uncommunicative, and aloof, changes that sometimes can be attributed to mood swings.
- **Low self-esteem** Unless they are educated differently, individuals may misinterpret their illness behavior as a function of their own personality and be unnecessarily hard on themselves (self-condemning).
- **Destructive, "hair trigger" behavior** During a normal mood state, an individual might be a very conservative decision-maker. During a manic state, the same person can become reckless and hot-headed, endangering the lives of strangers and/or loved ones.

Unless they occur secondary to another illness, mood disorders are genetically determined. As mentioned earlier, hormonal shifts, psychological stress, other illnesses and seasonal changes tend to destabilize underlying depressive vulnerabilities. (Appendices F and G present case studies of major depression secondary to multiple sclerosis and major depression secondary to dementia.) For example, hormonal stress at menarche (beginning of menses) may trigger the onset of a mood disorder, or the period following childbirth may trigger postpartum "blues" or depression. Menopausal stress may trigger late-onset or recurrent depression. Cyclical depressive episodes of this type usually last 3 to 9 months.

Each of the primary mood disorders affects awareness in a unique way. Major depression produces a dysphoric state, meaning that subjective awareness always is painful. Most of the illness behavior associated with depression intersects the awareness center. There are occasions, however, when patients may appear improved—as is the case when patients improve with the use of antidepressants—before they are aware of any improvement.[16]

Manic states tend to produce behavior that bypasses awareness. Patients may experience euphoria during a manic episode (behavior that reflects a positive cognitive assignment to the mood state) or dysphoria (behavior that reflects a negative cognitive assignment to the mood state). During mixed states, all behavior intersects awareness. Patients display signs of both depression and mania, and their behavior usually is marked by severe agitation, psychosis and dysphoria.

Beyond the three primary classifications of depression, mania, and mixed state, mood disorders can be further differentiated as either unipolar or bipolar. Unipolar patients have only one possible "pole" (expression) of their illness, i.e., depression. Bipolar patients have two possible poles, i.e., depression and mania, but may manifest only one pole of illness, often leading to confusion of diagnosis. (Appendices H and I present case studies of bipolar and unipolar depression.)

The symptoms of depression are the same for unipolar and bipolar depression. Although there is no definitive way to determine the presence of either condition, except when there is a positive history of mania, the following trends can be helpful in establishing more conclusive identification:

Unipolar Trends	Bipolar Trends
Later onset of illness (age 45)	Earlier onset of illness (age 25)
Little family history	Loaded family history
Negative postpartum depression	Positive postpartum depression
Negative antidepressant induced hypomania (mania)	Positive antidepressant induced hypomania (mania)
Agitation with somatic complaints	Hypersomnolence/ increased appetite
Few cycles in a lifetime	Many cycles in a lifetime (lifetime average is 4)

The evolution of bipolar disorder may be related to the behavioral adaptability of hypomania.[17] Hypomania is characterized by increased energy, increased optimism, and sharpened thinking. Progression of bipolar disorder to maladaptive levels may have been limited in the past by the average life span, which—until 1900—was approximately 45 years of age.

In general, major depression and mania are opposite types of behavior, with depression representing underactivation of brain function and mania representing overactivation of brain function. As mentioned earlier, both mood disorders can be identified by analysis of behavioral clusters, the signs and symptoms that differentiate depressed or manic patients from patients with other types of disorders. The following table demonstrates criteria for the opposite poles of major depression and hypomania:

Criteria for Hypomania	Criteria for Major Depression
Euphoria, inflated self-esteem	Dysphoria, depressed mood
Decreased need for sleep	Insomnia or hypersomnia (increased sleep)
Talkativeness, racing thoughts	Psychomotor agitation, retardation (slowed thinking)
Distractability	Diminished thinking (inability to complete or focus on one task)
Increase in goal-oriented activity (high motivation)	Fatigue, loss of energy (low motivation)
Excessive involvement in pleasureable activities or increased capacity to experience pleasure	Diminished interest or decreased capacity to experience pleasure

Proper identification and treatment of mood disorders is critical because of the life-threatening nature of these illnesses.[18] Unfortunately, nonrecognition and misdiagnosis are common[19] and occur for many reasons:

1. Our society's failure to legitimize physical disorders affecting the brain
2. The tendency to seek help from professionals (i.e., internists, sleep and sexual dysfunction experts, therapists, pastors, and priests) who do not specialize in the treatment of mood disorders
3. Lack of accurate information for the general public about mood disorders

Diagnosis of mood disorders involves a series of physical and neurologic examinations, which are performed to rule out physical illnesses that might cause depressive syndromes or interfere with treatment responses. Included in the examinations are:

1. Electroencephalogram (EEG)
2. Urinalysis (U/A)
3. Blood chemistries (SMA-C)
4. Complete blood count (CBC)
5. Vitamin B-12 and folate levels
6. Thyroid profile with TSH (thyroid stimulating hormone) and possible TRH (thyroid releasing hormone) challenge

Family history of mood disorders or other psychiatric disorders also is researched. History of medical illnesses is examined, as many can produce psychiatric symptoms. Strokes, for example, can produce biological depression. In addition, prescription medications that are being taken for illnesses and illicit drugs must be considered as possible contributing factors to mood disorders.

Anxiety Disorders

Summary: Anxiety disorders are characterized by a subjective sense of being anxious and a heightened state of nervous system arousal. Disorders included in this category are panic disorder, generalized anxiety disorder (GAD), posttraumatic stress disorder (PTSD), and conversion disorder. Panic disorders are determined mainly by intrinsic mechanisms within the brain that create anxiety. GAD, PTSD, and conversion disorder are determined primarily by extrinsic mechanisms.

Panic Disorder[21] is caused by a defect in the brain stem mechanism ("on-off" switch) that controls response to perceived danger. The "on-off" switch can be activated on random occasions or under the influence of stress, resulting in severe and debilitating panic attacks.

The neuromechanical foundation for panic disorder is based on hypersensitive cellular response. In individuals who have this condition, a lower-than-average amount of neurotransmitter is produced in everyday situations, creating cells that are "up-regulated" and unstable. On those occasions when a normal amount of neurotransmitter is released, cells become overreactive and trigger a panic attack.

A panic attack is an adaptation of the normal "fight or flight" survival mechanism seen throughout the animal kingdom. For example, during the prehistoric era when early man was confronted by a snarling saber-toothed tiger, a form of panic attack took place, the "do or die" response (characterized by elevated heart and respiratory rate), which increases chances of survival. The actual symptoms of a panic attack are viewed as normal in the presence of real danger but can become very destructive in the absence of true threat.

Panic attacks occur without warning and with very severe effects, somewhat like being hit over the head from behind with a two-by-four. Generally, there are four phases through which attacks progress:

1. The attack is defined by its **DSM-IV criteria**
2. **Anticipatory anxiety** occurs secondary to the attack
3. **Avoidance behavior** is present
4. **Demoralization** (feelings of depression and hopelessness) set in

The horror of the randomness with which panic attacks strike cannot be underestimated. For example, mice that are shocked at a highly predictable rate cope with the shock well. When the same mice are shocked without warning, they become severely agitated and dysfunctional. The intensity of the human response to panic attacks frequently is heightened by the random quality; as attack frequency increases, the intensity of anticipatory anxiety grows and can reach a point where it is constant and so severe that patients no longer can recognize the occurrence of an attack.[22] If the emotional and psychological pain is too great after the onset of demoralization, suicide may result. In fact, suicide *does* occur in approximately 20 percent of all panic disorder cases.

Treatment of panic disorders is focused on keeping the brain stem mechanism (the "on-off" switch) that regulates response to threat or danger, in the "off" position. Double-blind studies have shown that certain medications aid this effort. As is true with classical conditioning, the phase of inappropriate response (i.e., anticipatory anxiety and avoidance behavior) slowly dissipates; patients begin to experience a lengthy period of desensitization that is much like learning to set aside the anticipation of being hit over the head with a two-by-four.

General Anxiety Disorder[23] is characterized by anxiety and apprehensive expectation (worry). It can occur at any age, but is most often seen in childhood and adolescence. Instead of occurring in discrete periods (as with panic attacks), GAD occurs continuously. Stress in the environment causes the reticular activating system (RAS) to increase its output, and the ongoing anxiety that is present in response to stress causes apprehensive expectation. For example, an individual who has just received notification from the IRS that his many bogus investments do not qualify for tax deductions is a perfect candidate for GAD, as he probably will experience severe anxiety about financial loss and possible bankruptcy. A prolonged divorce proceeding also can trigger GAD.

With regard to considering content of life as a major contributor to illness, GAD is an exception to the rule. Treatment involves support groups, counseling to develop solutions for stressors and anxiety medications.

The adaptive function of GAD is preparing the brain to deal with the threat of stress. Maintaining normal amounts of alertness and heightened vigilance ensures greater chances of survival. Excessive alertness, however, can lead to impairment and maladaptive behavior. GAD usually develops in the following stages:

Stage 1 Stress produces constant anxiety
Stage 2 Anxiety produces worry about stress

Posttraumatic Stress Disorder[24] is a memory disorder created by severe stress-induced anxiety; it can occur at any age.[25] Presumably, PTSD mechanisms originally evolved for useful purposes, such as reminding prehistoric man that if a particular event had been life-threatening in the recent past, it still could have the same effect in the near future.

Group support therapy can be helpful for PTSD patients, and medical therapy targets the features of PTSD, i.e., anxiety/avoidance behavior, depression, and GAD. There is no known medical therapy to correct the memory disturbance itself.

Normal memory involves a specific event ("fact memory") and the time of the event ("episodic memory"). "Recollection of stored information refers to the conscious recall of previously learned information . . . ."[26]

The development of PTSD unfolds in phases that correspond to the DSM-IV criteria for PTSD:

Stage A Onset of **acute stress, anxiety and agitation** in response to traumatic event corresponds to criterion no. 1.

Stage B **Memory disturbance** corresponds to criterion no. 2.

Stage C **Avoidance behavior** corresponds to criterion no. 3.

1. efforts to avoid thoughts
2. efforts to avoid activities
3. inability to recall

Demoralization or depression
4. decreased interest
5. feelings of detachment
6. restricted range of affect

Stage D Development of **generalized anxiety disorder** (GAD) corresponds to criterion no. 4.

1. difficulty falling asleep
2. irritability
3. decreased ability to concentrate
4. hypervigilance
5. exaggerated startle response

Stage "A" for PTSD involves a severe threat, which causes intense fear and anxiety. In children, it may be exhibited as agitation. The "B," "C," and "D" stages are consequences of the "A" stage.

Stage "B" describes consequences of abnormal memory function. Normal recall involves executive function initiating recall or memories. PTSD involves recurrent and intrusive distress with recollection of a particular event, including images, thoughts, or perceptions.

Recurrent images of PTSD can be confused with perceptual disturbances of a traditional psychosis. The abnormal memory

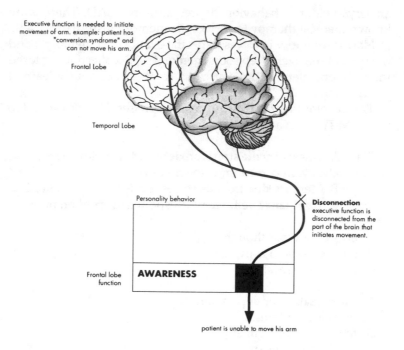

Executive function is needed to initiate
movement of arm. example: patient has
"conversion syndrome" and
can not move his arm.

Frontal Lobe

Temporal Lobe

Personality behavior

Disconnection
executive function is
disconnected from the
part of the brain that
initiates movement.

Frontal lobe   **AWARENESS**
function

patient is unable to move his arm

Figure 6-1. Temporary disconnection syndrome.

formation in PTSD causes awake memories to be experienced in instances where memories normally are not experienced. They also occur spontaneously or intrusively. Typically, a memory contains *information* about an event although individuals do not *experience* the event.

The brain *does* provide means by which a memory can be experienced—through dreams. With PTSD, memories are experienced during the awake state and dreams are experienced as horrible nightmares.

Acting or feeling as if the traumatic event is recurring may be created by a mechanism that is similar to a pseudoseizure, where patients reenact a trauma-specific event. Reminders of the event can trigger intense distress or physiologic reactivity.

In summary, PTSD follows a sequence that begins with a traumatic event, moves on to memory disturbance, progresses to depression/demoralization or avoidance behavior, and finally leads to generalized anxiety.

Temporary Disconnection Syndrome

At the Biological Psychiatry Institute and in this text, the term "temporary disconnection syndrome" (TDS) replaces the term "conversion syndrome" used in the DSM-IV. My professional experience and research lead me to believe that conversion syndrome is a neuropsychiatric syndrome caused by frontal lobe dysfunction. I have renamed it because the new title more accurately describes the temporary disconnection of executive function from other parts of the brain.

From a psychodynamic point of view "conversion syndrome" implies that internal conflicts within the brain are "converted" into physical symptoms. Virtually no psychodynamic theory has yielded a valid neuropsychiatric disorder. For instance, schizophrenia and obsessive compulsive disorder once were viewed as being caused by inappropriate toilet training by parents. It is now known that schizophrenia is a valid neuropsychiatric disorder secondary to abnormal migration of neurons and that obsessive compulsive disorder is strongly genetically determined Depression was thought to be a result of subconscious conflicts but today susceptibility to depression is known to be hereditary.

TDS occurs when abnormal behavior is temporarily produced, which does not conform with usual anatomical outlines or behavioral patterns. This takes place when frontal lobes of the brain (the final common pathway for brain input and output) are temporarily disconnected from other areas of the brain. The disorder involves temporary disconnection of executive function from awareness. Executive function controls the shift of attention between various areas of awareness and selects behavioral output, which can range from initiating motor movement, the execution of working memory or the retrieval of memory.

Clinical presentations of TDS include temporary paralysis, unusual sensory defects, pseudoseizures (complex motor activity that resembles a seizure but is not caused by spontaneous discharges of the brain), and the presence of multiple personalities (when an individual acts like someone else)

Specific examples of TDS follow.

It has been observed that TDS patients are more easily hypnotized than other individuals. For instance, those with pseudoseizures can be hypnotized into initiating or ending a "seizure." Under hypnosis some individuals can completely disconnect the sensation of pain from their awareness. In fact, major surgeries have been performed, pain-free, using hypnotism.

"Hysterical blindness" is another example of awareness that has disconnected from sensory input. Visual fields normally take on predictable patterns of perception, but altered awareness may produce visual patterns that do not conform to "anatomical patterns." Blindness (nonawareness) occurs temporarily and all visual reflexes are preserved.

"Hysterical paralysis" occurs when executive function cannot initiate movement. Again, paralysis is temporary and all reflex movements are preserved.

So-called multiple personalities occur when individuals involuntarily assume the characteristics of other people. "Acting"—assuming the traits of others, from a dramatic

---

Temporary Disconnection Syndrome *continued*

standpoint—is a type of complex behavior that occurs separately from the "real" personality but is voluntary.

Neurologists have coined the term "pseudoseizure" to designate behavior that mimics a true seizure. Like other types of TDS, pseudoseizures are caused by the release of complex motor acts that are controlled by frontal lobe executive function.

Some individuals are born with a hereditary predisposition toward TDS and others acquire the illness secondary to another disorder, such as multiple sclerosis. Since TDS is not permanent, the therapy used with patients who have this condition includes reassurance and, frequently, referral for psychotherapy. As is the case for *all* types of illness, stress may trigger TDS. When patients exhibit maladaptive behavior that creates excessive stress related to TDS, then psychotherapy is indicated. Continued vigilance for secondary causes of TDS must be maintained.

Many neurologists who are consulted by patients with TDS can find nothing wrong because presenting symptoms do not involve "usual" anatomical or behavioral patterns. On the other hand, patients with TDS who are seen at the Biological Psychiatry Institute are advised that their unusual condition is due to a problem with executive function. They are reassured that the disorder will resolve in time, when executive function reconnects. In some medical circles, however, there is a common perception of patients with TDS that they are not ill but are acting "crazy" or are simply malingering. In such environments it is not unusual for patients to be humiliated by diagnoses, such as "withdrawal reflexes are present," that "prove" nothing is wrong.

The symptoms of TDS—sudden paralysis, seizures, sudden numbness, sudden visual problems—can present a challenge to neurologists because such physical problems also can represent neurological emergencies or the presence of serious neurological disease (Clearly, more research is needed in this area.) Neurologists are obligated to rule out "organic" illness before they can make the diagnosis of "conversion syndrome" (TDS). Unfortunately, organic illness and conversion syndrome frequently occur simultaneously. As many as 40 percent of patients who have pseudoseizures also experience "real" seizures. This is not surprising because individuals with stored memories of "real" seizures are more likely to exhibit this behavior than those who have never experienced seizures.

Neurologists usually anguish over the diagnosis of a seizure versus a pseudoseizure because the two types of disorders occur together and are difficult to tell apart. Pseudoseizures may be treated *similarly* to panic attacks (as abnormal release phenomena), but many neurologists treat them in the same way, which often results in excessive use of medications and unnecessary hospitalizations. A better understanding of TDS is needed so that appropriate diagnoses and treatment plans can be made for disorders caused by TDS.

Conversion Disorder[27] is also known as Temporary Disconnection Syndrome (TDS), and typically occurs between the ages of 10 and

35, affecting voluntary control of motor or sensory function. This may be manifested as sudden paralysis of an arm or sudden inability to see. Psychological factors are thought to be the cause of conversion disorder. Specifically, stress causes certain vulnerable individuals to temporarily disconnect parts of their brain. (See Fig. 6-1 and "Temporary Disconnection Syndrome" on pages 117–118).

The DSM-IV criteria are self-explanatory but should be interpreted within the temporary disconnection syndrome. The sensory and motor deficits of this syndrome resolve on their own, so that supportive therapy is indicated.

Following are the developmental stages of conversion disorder:

Stage 1 Biologically vulnerable individual
Stage 2 Severe anxiety caused by extreme stress
Stage 3 Temporary disconnection (i.e., conversion)
Stage 4 Spontaneous remission

Obsessive Compulsive Disorders (OCD)

Summary: Caused by dysfunction in the basal ganglia and frontal lobes, OCD creates a release phenomenon involving **basic instincts** such as excessive handwashing (instinct to be clean), exaggerated lock-checking (instinct to maintain territoriality), and excessive hair pulling (grooming instinct). Eating disorders, which are caused by dysfunction in the hypothalamus, also are included in this category. These involve eating drives and mating (sexual) instincts that affect the way individuals perceive their own bodies.

Obsessive compulsive disorder[28] is an excessive release of instinctual behavior, resulting in obsessive thoughts and compulsions; usually, it is first seen in adolescence or early adulthood. Treatment for OCD involves medication to decrease the obsessive generator and/or systematic desensitization to obsessive thoughts.

Following is a listing of normal instincts and the abnormal behavior that is produced in the presence of OCD.

Instinct to be clean	Obsessive thoughts of contamination hands and clean	Compulsion to wash
Territorial instinct	Obsessive thoughts about breach of territoriality	Compulsion to check locks
Bonding instinct	Obsessive thoughts about infidelity	Compulsion to stalk

Grooming instinct	Obsessive thoughts about hair	Compulsive hair-pulling
Instinct to preserve survival materials	Obsessive thoughts about obtaining materials	Compulsive hoarding
Instinct to Organize	Obsessive thoughts about orderliness	Compulsion for symmetry
Sexual instinct	Obsessive thoughts about sex	Sexual compulsions

In the presence of OCD, tension builds until a particular instinctual thought is satisfied. Rituals may temporarily satisfy the obsessive thoughts. As has been observed with instinctive generators, obsessive generators are powerful determinants of behavior and require repeated counteractive inputs to avoid severe subjective tension.

If an instinct is satisfied, the result is great pleasure. Conversely, if an instinct is unfulfilled, dysphoria results. With OCD, the pain of not satisfying an obsession is severe dysphoria so OCD patients almost always do what they can to satisfy their obsessions. It is not unusual, for example, for OCD patients to spend several hours a day repeating rituals.

All illnesses have the potential for obsessiveness. For instance, a schizophrenic may be obsessively concerned that the FBI is listening to private telephone conversations. A depressed patient may become obsessively aware of a specific negative thought. A panic patient may become obsessed with anticipatory anxiety. Therefore, in order to make an accurate diagnosis of OCD, other illnesses that can cause obsessiveness first must be ruled out. (Appendix J presents a case study of Masked OCD; Appendix K describes Juvenile OCD).

Several classifications of OCD will be briefly discussed here: social phobia, body dysmorphic disorder (BDD), hypochondriasis, somatization disorder, pain disorder, and eating disorders. These disorders are included in the OCD classification because their symptoms are produced by release of an instinctive generator of behavior.

Social Phobia[29] involves the social instinct of being watched and judged by others, but in this case, the normal instinct is expressed obsessively. The subjective assignment to social phobic thoughts is severe anxiety and fear. Although patients are aware that the obsessive thoughts are unreasonable, anxiety and fear cause them to avoid social situations.

Body Dysmorphic Disorder[30] is involved with how individuals instinctively perceive themselves. Self-perception is awareness of the internal world, accompanied by subjective assignments. BDD causes obsessive thoughts about a suspected defect in appearance. Patients with this disorder frequently request plastic surgery.

Hypochondriasis[31] is a preoccupation (based on misinterpretation of physical symptoms) with fears of having a serious disease. Because the threshold for assigning a subjective state to illness is very low, patients experience the obsessive and distressing sensation of having a critical illness.

Somatization Disorder[32] involves the instinct to integrate and feel pain. Instead of a normal general threshold for a subjective assignment for pain, the threshold for pain integration in the thalamus is low. (Since all sensory input is integrated in the thalamus, one would expect a general sensory dysfunction syndrome.) Although there is no medical condition to account for pain, the patient experiences pain in a diffuse manner. Four specific characteristics suggest a somatization disorder:

1. Involvement of multiple organ systems
2. Early onset/chronic course
3. No physical signs to account for pain or laboratory abnormalities to indicate illness
4. Patient does not feign symptoms

Pain Disorder is a common syndrome, as can be seen by the many pain clinics that have developed throughout the United States in recent years. The DSM-IV criteria for pain disorder[33] are self-explanatory. A result of normal integration of pain and normal subjective assignment to pain, pain disorder arises from increased sensory input originating with a real source.

For example, in the case of chronic back pain, the increased sensory signals from the spine and related areas can result in obsessive thoughts about pain; if these thoughts cannot be controlled, formalized pain disorder ensues. Pain disorder syndrome is difficult to treat because normal mechanisms are involved, and a multimodel treatment approach (as utilized in pain clinics) typically must be used.

Eating Disorders are characterized by eating behavioral disturbances and usually present in three primary forms—bulimia nervosa, anorexia nervosa, and obesity.[32] As is true with all obsessive compulsive disorders, individuals with eating disorders are normal except for their obsessive thoughts (in this case, as they relate to eating).

Bulimia Nervosa[35] usually is categorized as binge eating with compensatory behavior, such as self-induced vomiting, excessive exercise, or use of laxatives.

The first stage of bulimia, which normally begins in adolescence and is more prevalent in females than in males,[36] is comprised of obsessive thoughts about eating, i.e., release of the eating instinct. If patients do not heed bulimic thoughts, they are flooded with overwhelming anxiety, which they feel even before eating.

The second stage involves extreme dysphoria in relation to excessive eating and also relates to the subjective assignment made by our culture (the content of society) that "Thin is sexy and fat is ugly." Presumably, if a culture transmitted the message, "The fatter you are, the better you look," bulimia would have only one stage within a social context.

During the second stage patients try to eliminate absorption of calories by vomiting, using laxatives or exercising heavily. Medical complications include:

- Death from heart failure (prolonged use of syrup of ipecac can cause heart failure)
- Loss of teeth (from repeated exposure to stomach acid)
- Pancreatitis
- Stomach ulcers
- Suicide
- Malnutrition and associated disorders

Medical treatment for bulimia nervosa involves blocking the obsessive compulsive thoughts about eating.

Anorexia Nervosa[37] is a severe internal perceptual disorder, which commonly presents around age 17, and results in dysphoria with loss of appetite. The condition reflects learned social values that "fat is bad." There is no adequate treatment at this time.

The DSM-IV criteria for anorexia provides another example of psychiatric bias when one diagnostic criterion states that individuals with this disorder *choose* to refuse to maintain body weight. In fact, medical disorders of the brain are not disorders of will or self-control; anorexia patients are *unable* to maintain body weight.

One of the criterion for anorexia—"intense fear of gaining weight or becoming fat, even though underweight"—defines this disorder as being one of anticipatory anxiety leading to fear.

Anorexia patients project into the future and experience the dysphoria of being fat. Depressed patients, on the other hand, experience no anticipatory anxiety because, for them, "There is no future." Panic patients reflect anticipatory anxiety related to future events. The subjective sense of time is affected by many brain disorders.

The criterion that notes a disturbance in the way in which anorexic patients experience their body weight and shape reflects inaccurate self-evaluation. The disturbance of experience could be interpreted as a traditional psychosis (i.e., circumscribed disorder of experience or perceptual disturbance). Typically the awareness center is flooded with thoughts of illness, and patients hold fixed beliefs (circumscribed delusions) that they are fat, in spite of appearing emaciated. Patients *believe* they are overweight and actually *experience* sensations associated with being overweight.

Schizophrenic Disorders

Summary: These disorders are caused by a combination of temporal lobe overactivity (producing delusions or hallucinations) and/or frontal lobe underactivity (producing blunted affect and social isolation).

Viewed primarily as a traditional psychosis with frontal dysfunction, schizophrenia[38] is not caused by a definable source, such as hallucinogenic drugs or depression. This class of disorders is believed to be related to developmental migration of brain cells.[39] The resulting abnormality causes inhibition of frontal lobe functioning (i.e., flattening of affect, loss of executive function or disorganized behavior) and excitation of temporal lobe function (i.e., auditory hallucinations). *Negative symptoms* of schizophrenia refer to elements that inhibit the frontal lobes. *Positive symptoms* refer to elements that activate the temporal lobes. Treatment involves reversing the two above-described processes.

The subtypes of schizophrenic disorders relate to the dominant lobe in the brain that is affected by schizophrenia. *Paranoid types* relate to temporal lobe dysfunction characterized by:

- Delusions, or disorders of belief
- Hallucinations, or disorders of perception
- Disorganized speech, or disorders of language

Disorganized types relate to frontal lobe dysfunction characterized by:

- Grossly disorganized or catatonic behavior
- Negative symptoms

Catatonic types relate to frontal lobe dysfunction with diffuse brain dysfunction.

Cognitive deficits associated with schizophrenia are less appreciated.

Attention Deficit Disorder (ADD)

Summary: Characterized by inattentiveness, poor planning ability, and impaired capacity to execute and follow through on tasks, ADD is the result of too little right frontal lobe function (i.e., working memory).

Attention deficit disorder (ADD) is a common brain disorder that usually presents in childhood, does not dissipate in adolescence, and is common in more than 5 percent of adults. It may or may not be associated with hyperactivity, and typical symptoms for both children and adults include poor attention, hyperactivity, and impulsivity. The neuropsychiatric deficit is in the frontal lobes (primarily on the right side) and involves working memory, a temporary memory buffer that allows individuals to plan and synthesize information. Because ADD patients have difficulty applying their intelligence, knowledge, and experience, they are underachievers. Frequently, they are perceived as lazy or lacking motivation.[40] Treatment involves the use of psychostimulants.

A summary of Chapters 6 and 7 is provided at the end of Chapter 7.

References

1. No brain disorders are classified as "minor."
2. A brain disorder usually is identified by the dominant feature or generator of behavior, such as major depression. Sometimes, on initial presentation, patients' concerns involve secondary generators of behavior, such as sexual dysfunction, insomnia, chronic fatigue, and pain syndrome. Therefore, when patients present in specialty clinics, it is important to screen for an underlying, primary etiology.

   Research and scientific findings with regard to major brain disorders have come in phases, each one accompanied by a major drug discovery:

1970	Mood disorders	Lithium
1980	Anxiety disorders	Tricyclic antidepressants
1990	Obsessive compulsive disorders	SSRI
1990 2000	Schizophrenia	Atypical antipsychotics

3. "Personality" behavior implies that:

   - Activities are part of the normal behavioral matrix called "personality"
   - Activities are present or potentially present at all times
   - Activities are part of the total feedback mechanism that represents control, as opposed to being independent generators of behavior that represent illness
   - Activities are subject to will and self-control via executive function

4. The usefulness of psychotherapy is well established in treating mild depression when psychosocial stressors are present. At one time it was believed that psychotherapy also was effective for moderate or severe depression, but this benefit now is known to be largely illusory. The perceived improvement in severe symptoms generally coincided with spontaneous remission of depression that naturally occurs 3 to 9 months after the onset of depression.

5. As of this writing, neuropsychiatry is not yet a formally recognized medical subspecialty but is being practiced by a handful of medical practitioners in this country and around the world.

6. Genetically determined brain disorders probably are related to the evolutionary process. For instance, the manic part of manic depressive illness originally may have had an adaptable function in allowing creative genius to manifest itself over a brief period of time. Then, if an individual were a victim of war, famine, or disease, creativity still would have a chance to be expressed. In the case of obsessive compulsive disorder, the instinct to be clean (i.e., repetitive handwashing) may have had an adaptable function in preventing the spread of disease.

7. Before the availability of medications, mood disorders tended to worsen with age. In fact, mood cycles occurred more frequently and the depth of depression was greater.

8. Although family history is the main information source about DNA, we do not yet have the technology to define genetic or primary brain disorders by direct examination of DNA.

9. We *do* know that when the limbic system cuts across generators of behavior involving the frontal lobes, hypothalamus, and temporal lobes, clusters of depressive symptoms (as defined in DSM-IV) are produced. For instance, a patient may have a sleep or appetite problem that occurs within the context of a major depressive syndrome. Other

generators of behavior at times may be vulnerable to limbic system dysfunction, producing variations of major depression (i.e., anxious depression, obsessoid depression, psychotic depression).

Below are listed the symptoms of major depression, according to the region in the brain where each originates and the purpose of that specific region:

Symptom	Brain Region	Purpose
Depressed mood	Limbic lobe	Controls mood
Diminished interest	Hypothalamus	Controls pleasure
Weight loss or gain	Hypothalamus	Controls appetite
Insomnia or hypersomnia	Hypothalamus	Controls sleep
Psychomotor agitation	Frontal lobes	Control motor activity
Fatigue	Hypothalamus	Controls energy levels
Feelings of worthlessness	Temporal lobes	Control sense of self-esteem
Diminished ability to concentrate	Frontal lobes	Control ability to concentrate
Recurrent thoughts of death	Temporal lobes	Control instinct to live

10. The firing rate of a cell is the number of electrical impulses that travel down the axon leading to the release of neurotransmitters. Stimulation of neuroreceptors (as a result of neurotransmitters) can result in a depolarization potential or an electrical impulse that travels down the axon of a brain cell. The density of neuroreceptors affects the firing rate of the brain cell.

11. "Kindling" in the brain is like lighting a forest fire. Once the fire is ignited and begins to spread, it is difficult to control, and the forest is forever changed. In the same way, the longer patients who are vulnerable to schizophrenic and manic-depressive illness experience active illness, the further their illness (the "fire") progresses. Medical science is more effective in *preventing* active illness than in *treating* active symptoms.

    Kindling also applies to juvenile brain physiology. If children who are genetically vulnerable to violent behavior are nurtured in a peaceful environment, they will tend to be nonviolent. If these same children are subjected to a violent environment, they will be subject to a biological kindling effect. A violent environment will tend to bring out violent behavior, which will tend to be continuous.

    Currently, biological psychiatric treatment strategies involve controlling psychotic episodes in schizophrenia and mood swings in manic-depressive illness. Violent behavior is controlled by providing social programs that promote peaceful environments. In the future, through genetic engineering (that actually changes genetic material in the neuron), strategies will involve pretreatment of children and adolescents—before active symptoms appear—in order to prevent illness.

12. The DSM-IV (p. 327) gives the following criteria ("behavioral cluster") for Major Depressive Syndrome:

- depressed mood
- diminished interest in activities
- significant weight loss or gain
- insomnia or hypersomnia
- psychomotor agitation or retardation
- fatigue
- feelings of excessive guilt
- diminished ability to concentrate
- recurrent thoughts of death or suicide

When determining the presence of depression, the above characteristics must be taken into consideration as well as the following elements:

- Did the depression occur for no apparent reason?
- Is the depression pervasive? If clinical depression truly is present, there is no distraction from feeling depressed. For instance, individuals may feel depressed in the morning after paying bills or arguing with family members, but in the afternoon the same individuals may enjoy a baseball game or going shopping. Clinically depressed patients find their mood all-encompassing and are unable to enjoy any type of activity.
- Has the patient had similar episodes that responded to medication? Except for side effects, antidepressants have no impact on normal behavior. When a patient responds to medication, this has both diagnostic and therapeutic meaning. The diagnostic meaning is that the patient has a medical disorder; the therapeutic meaning is that the patient responds to a particular medication.

13. Depressed patients have no capacity to enjoy anything in the *present*, including friends, food, and hobbies. There is no capacity to appreciate the *past*, and memories are accompanied by constant feelings of guilt. Sense about the *future* is dim and characterized by hopelessness. Sleep or restful sleep is impossible and patients suffer deep pain over being sleep-deprived.

Since there is no relief in the past, present, future, or in sleep, depressed patients only can experience pain. They usually feel isolated and misunderstood because no one else can "see" their pain; friends and family members may advise those who are depressed to "shake it off" or to "pull yourself up by the bootstraps." Consequently, unless patients receive appropriate treatment, suicide is a high risk.

14. Manic and hypomanic states manifest the same symptoms although they affect functioning differently. Mania, the more extreme degree of activation, drastically affects function and may be associated with psychosis. Hypomania, on the other hand, has little effect on function and is not associated with psychosis.

The DSM-IV (p. 338) gives the following criteria for Hypomania:

- A distinct period of persistently elevated, expansive, or irritable mood, lasting throughout at least 4 days, that is clearly different from the usual nondepressed mood.
- During the period of mood disturbance, three (or more) of the following symptoms have persisted (four, if the mood is only irritable) and have been present to a significant degree:

    1. inflated self-esteem or grandiosity
    2. decreased need for sleep (i.e., feels rested after only 3 hours of sleep)
    3. more talkative than usual or pressure to keep talking
    4. flight of ideas or subjective experience that thoughts are racing
    5. distractability (i.e., attention too easily drawn to unimportant or irrelevant external stimuli)
    6. increase in goal-directed activity (either socially, at work or school, or sexually) or psychomotor agitation
    7. excessive involvement in pleasurable activities that have a high potential for painful consequences (i.e., the person engages in unrestrained buying sprees, sexual indiscretions, or foolish business investments)

- The episode is associated with an unequivocal change in functioning that is uncharacteristic of the person when not symptomatic.
- The disturbance in mood and the change in functioning are observable by others.
- The episode is not severe enough to cause marked impairment in social or occupational functioning, or to necessitate hospitalization, and there are no psychotic features.
- The symptoms are not due to the direct physiological effects of a substance (i.e., a drug of abuse, a medication or other treatment) or a general medical condition (i.e., hyperthyroidism).

15. Mixed states truly are a mixture of manic and depressive symptoms. An individual in a mixed state might say, "While I was decorating my house last night, I also was planning my suicide." Note that the manic activation is reflected in the act of decorating the house, while a depressive state is reflected in planning a suicide.

16. This difference in perception is illustrated in nurses' notes that describe patient improvement and patients' notes for the same time period that lack any described improvement. When I note improvement in my own patients but they do not feel improved, I reassure them that their *apparent* improvement predicts that they will *feel* improved with time.

17. "Mania" and "hypomania" are terms that refer to a degree of brain activation. Mania is severe and implies that psychiatric hospitalization is needed. Hypomania is a milder form of brain activation that usually does not require hospitalization.

18. Suicide is a severe risk with major depression and mixed states. In the case of manic disorders, noncompliance (failure to take mood stabilizing medications) can lead to loss of job and/or friends, antisocial behavior, financial loss, accidental injury, or death. Mania also can accelerate into catatonia, which eventually can require hospitalization and can be fatal.

    Suicidal thoughts reflect a particular brain capacity, which can be activated in three different ways:

    • *rational thought* occurs when an individual is in extreme pain, near death and wants to die with dignity.
    • *content of life* may cause certain coping mechanisms that may be adaptive or maladaptive, such as a "cry for help" or a suicidal gesture by someone overwhelmed by stress.
    • *illness behavior* occurs independent of personality structure and may be lethal; because it is not subject to will or self-control, illness behavior is the most dangerous origin for suicidal thoughts.

19. More than 6 percent of Americans suffer from some form of mood disorder, but only one-third of these receive treatment.

20. Use of the following medications (*Journal of Clinical Psychiatry* 1986;47[1, suppl]:3–9) frequently is associated with the occurrence of mood disorders:

Class and Generic Name	Trade Name
Antihypertensives	
Reserpine	Serpasil, Ser-Ap-Es, Sandril
Methyldopa	Aldomet
Propranolol hydrochloride	Inderal
Guanethidine sulfate	Ismelin sulfate

| Hydralazine hydrochloride | Spresoline hydrochloride |
| Clonidine hydrochloride | Catapres |

Antiparkinsonian Agents
Levodopa	Dopar, Laradopa
Levodopa and carbidopa	Sinemet
Amantadine hydrochloride	Symmetrel

Hormones
| Estrogen | Evex, Menrium |
| Progesterone | Lipo-Lutin, Prolution |

Corticosteroids
| Cortisone acetate | Cortone Acetate |

Antituberculosis
| Cycloserine | Seromycin |

Anticancer
| Vincristine sulfate | Oncovin |
| Vinblastine sulfate | Velban |

21. The DSM-IV (p. 395) gives the following criteria for Panic Disorder (panic attack). Typically, individuals with panic disorder will abruptly develop at least 4 out of the 13 named criteria, which will reach maximum intensity within a 10-minute period:

   • palpitations, pounding heart or accelerated heart rate
   • sweating
   • trembling or shaking
   • sensations of shortness of breath or smothering
   • feeling of choking
   • chest pain or discomfort
   • nausea or abdominal distress
   • feeling dizzy, unsteady, lightheaded or faint
   • derealization (feelings of unreality) or depersonalization (being detached from oneself)
   • fear of losing control or going crazy
   • fear of dying
   • paresthesias (numbness or tingling sensations)
   • chills or hot flushes

   It also may be helpful to list these symptoms according to the part of the body they affect:

1. Brain symptoms
   - fear of losing control or going crazy
   - fear of dying
   - derealization or depersonalization

2. Midline symptoms (chest/abdomen)
   - palpitations, pounding heart or accelerated heart rate
   - sensations of shortness of breath or smothering
   - feeling of choking
   - chest pain or discomfort
   - nausea or abdominal distress

3. Peripheral structure symptoms
   - sweating (usually hands)
   - trembling or shaking (usually in hands)
   - feeling dizzy, unsteady, lightheaded or faint
   - paresthesias (usually numbness in hands, feet, lips)
   - chills or hot flushes

22. When the anticipatory anxiety becomes so severe that the patient cannot leave home, the condition is called agoraphobia.

23. The DSM-IV (pp. 435–436) gives the following criteria for General Anxiety Disorder. Adult individuals must experience three or more symptoms, while only one is required for children:

   - restlessness or feeling on edge
   - becoming easily fatigued
   - difficulty concentrating or mind going blank
   - irritability
   - muscle tension
   - sleep disturbance

24. The DSM-IV (pp. 427–429) gives the following criteria for Posttraumatic Stress Disorder:

   - The individual experienced, witnessed, or was confronted with an event or events that involved actual or threatened death or serious injury, or a threat to the physical integrity of self or others.
   - The traumatic event is persistently reexperienced in one or more of the following ways:

     1. recurrent, intrusive, distressing recollections of the event
     2. recurrent, distressing dreams of the event
     3. a sense of reliving the experience

4. intense distress upon exposure to cues that resemble an aspect of the traumatic event
5. physiological reactivity upon exposure to cues that resemble an aspect of the traumatic event

- Persistent avoidance of stimuli associated with the trauma and numbing of general responsiveness, as indicated by three or more of the following:

    1. efforts to avoid thoughts, feelings, or conversations associated with the trauma
    2. efforts to avoid activities, places or people that arouse memories of the trauma
    3. inability to recall an important aspect of the trauma
    4. diminished interest in significant activities
    5. feeling of detachment or estrangement from others
    6. restricted range of feelings
    7. sense of a foreshortened future

- Persistent symptoms of increased arousal, as indicated by two or more of the following:

    1. difficulty falling and staying asleep
    2. irritability or outbursts of anger
    3. difficulty concentrating
    4. hypervigilance
    5. exaggerated startle response
    6. disturbance lasts for more than one month.
    7. disturbance causes significant distress in social, occupational, or other important areas of functioning.

25. PTSD became well known after the Vietnam War. It took on a controversial aspect when it was found that many GIs had used illegal drugs to dull their sensitivity to the pain and violence of the war, and in so doing also had inadvertently decreased the likelihood of developing PTSD.
26. Cummings JL. Amnesia and disorders of memory. *Psychiatric Times* 1996;8(8):30.
27. The DSM-IV (p. 456) gives the following criteria for Conversion Disorder:

    - There are one or more symptoms affecting voluntary or sensory function.
    - Psychological factors are associated with the symptom because initiation of the symptom coincides with conflicts or other stressors.

- The symptom of deficit is not intentionally produced.
- The symptom cannot be fully explained by a general medical condition.
- The symptom causes sufficient distress to warrant medical evaluation.
- The symptom is not limited to pain or sexual dysfunction and is not better accounted for by another mental disorder.

28. The DSM-IV (pp. 422–423) gives the following criteria for Obsessive Compulsive Disorder:

Obsessions are defined as follows:
- recurrent, persistent thoughts (about real-life issues) that are intrusive and cause marked anxiety
- thoughts, impulses, or images are not simply excessive worries about real-life problems
- individual attempts to ignore or suppress such thoughts, impulses, or images, or to neutralize them with other thoughts or actions
- individual recognizes that the obsessional thoughts, impulses, or images are a product of his or her own mind

Compulsions are defined as follows:
- repetitive behaviors or mental acts that the individual feels driven to perform in response to an obsession or according to rules that must be applied rigidly
- the behaviors or mental acts are aimed at preventing or reducing distress or preventing some dreaded event or situation; however, these behaviors or mental acts either are not connected in a realistic way with what they are designed to neutralize or prevent or are clearly excessive
- At some point during the course of the disorder, the individual has recognized that the obsessions or compulsions are excessive or unreasonable (does not apply to children).
- The obsessions or compulsions cause marked distress, are time consuming (take more than one hour a day) or significantly interfere with the individual's normal routine, occupational (or academic) functioning, or usual social activities or relationships.
- If another Axis I disorder is present, the content of the obsessions or compulsions is not restricted to it (i.e., preoccupation with food in the presence of an Eating Disorder; hair pulling in the presence of Trichotillomania; concern with appearance in the presence of Body Dysmorphic Disorder; preoccupation with drugs in the presence of a Substance Use Disorder; preoccupation with having a serious illness in the presence of Hypochondriasis; preoccupation with sexual urges or fantasies

in the presence of a Paraphilia; or guilty ruminations in the presence of Major Depressive Disorder).

- The disturbance is not due to the direct physiological effects of a substance (i.e., a drug of abuse, a medication) or a general medical condition.

29. The DSM-IV (pp. 416 417) gives the following criteria for Social Phobia:

   - Marked, persistent fear of one or more social situations.
   - Fear of social situation may be expressed as a panic attack.
   - Individual recognizes that the fear is excessive and unreasonable.
   - Feared situations are avoided or endured with intense anxiety.
   - Avoidance and anxiety interfere significantly with normal routine.
   - For individuals younger than 18, duration is at least 6 months.
   - Avoidance and anxiety are not due to the direct physiologic effects of a substance or general medical condition.
   - If a general medical condition is present, anxiety and fear are unrelated to it.

30. The DSM-IV (p. 468) gives the following criteria for Body Dysmorphic Disorder:

   - Preoccupation with an imagined flaw in appearance.
   - Preoccupation causes clinically significant distress.
   - Preoccupation is not better accounted for by another mental disorder.

31. The DSM-IV (p. 465) gives the following criteria for Hypochondriasis:

   - Preoccupation with fears about having a serious disease.
   - Preoccupation persists despite appropriate medical evaluation.
   - Preoccupation is not of delusional intensity and not restricted to circumscribed concern about appearance.
   - Preoccupation causes clinically significant distress.
   - Duration of the disorder is at least 6 months.
   - Preoccupation is not better accounted for by any other disorder.

32. The DSM-IV (pp. 449–450) gives the following criteria for Somatization Disorder:

   - A history of many physical complaints, beginning before age 30, that occur over a period of several years and result in treatment being sought or significant impairment.

- Each of the following criteria must have been met during the course of the disturbance:

  1. four pain symptoms
  2. two gastrointestinal symptoms
  3. one sexual symptom
  4. one pseudoneurological symptom (the use of "pseudo-neurological" is an example of bias in psychiatry. This is actually a description of the disconnection syndrome. There is nothing "pseudo" [not authentic] about somatization disorder or any of the major brain disorders.

- Either of the following may be true:

  1. after appropriate investigation, each of the symptoms in Criterion B cannot be fully explained by a known general medical condition or the direct effects of a substance (i.e., a drug of abuse, a medication), or
  2. when there is a related general medical condition, the physical complaints or resulting social or occupational impairment are in excess of what would be expected from the history, physical examination or laboratory findings

- The symptoms are not intentionally produced or feigned (as in Factitious Disorder or Malingering).

33. The DSM-IV (p. 461) gives the following criteria for Pain Disorder:

- Pain in one or more anatomical site of sufficient severity to require clinical attention.
- Pain causes clinically significant distress or impairment in social, occupational or other important areas of functioning.
- Psychological factors are judged to have an important role in the onset, severity, exacerbation, or maintenance of pain.
- The symptom or deficit is not intentionally produced.
- Pain is not better accounted for by a mood, anxiety, or psychotic disorder.

34. Strictly speaking, obesity is considered a medical disorder because it is not consistently associated with an emotional syndrome. Obesity is included here as an eating disorder because of the multibillion dollar faddist industry that is based on the emotional *reaction* to obesity.

35. The DSM-IV (pp. 549–550) gives the following criteria for Bulimia Nervosa:

- Recurrent episodes of binge eating characterized by (1) eating within a discrete period of time an amount of food that is larger than most people would eat in the same period of time, or(2) a sense of a lack of control over eating.
- Recurrent inappropriate compensatory behavior designed to prevent weight gain, i.e., self-induced vomiting, misuse of laxatives, fasting, or excessive exercise.
- Binge eating and inappropriate compensatory behaviors occur at least twice a week for 3 months.
- Self-evaluation is unduly influenced by body shape and weight.
- The disturbance does not occur exclusively during episodes of anorexia nervosa.

36. Bulimia occurs in 1 to 3 percent of female adolescents and in 1/10-3/10 percent of males.
37. The DSM-IV (pp. 544–545) gives the following criteria for Anorexia Nervosa:

- Refusal to maintain body weight at or above a minimally normal weight for age and height.
- Intense fear of gaining weight or becoming fat, even though underweight.
- Disturbance in the way in which one's body weight or shape is experienced, undue influence of body weight/shape on self-evaluation or denial of the seriousness of current low body weight.
- In postmenstrual females, the absence of at least three consecutive menstrual cycles.

38. The DSM-IV (pp. 285–286) gives the following criteria for Schizophrenia:

- Two or more of the following symptoms, each present for a significant portion of time during a 1-month period: (a) delusions (b) hallucinations (c) disorganized speech (d) grossly disorganized or catatonic behavior, and (e) negative symptoms:
- One or more major areas of functioning, such as work and interpersonal relations, are markedly below the level achieved prior to the onset of symptoms.
- Continuous signs of the disturbance persist for at least 6 months.
- Schizoaffective disorder and mood disorder with psychotic features have been ruled out.
- Disturbance is not due to the direct physiological effects of a substance or general medical condition.
- If there is a history of autistic disorder or another pervasive developmental   disorder,   the   additional   diagnosis   of

schizophrenia is made only if prominent delusions or hallucinations also are present for at least 1 month.

39. In reality, schizophrenia involves the entire brain, as a result of abnormal neuronal migration that affects cognition and other capacities. As reflected in the diagnostic criteria, the diagnosis of schizophrenia traditionally focuses on frontal and temporal lobe dysfunction.

40. The DSM-IV (pp. 83–85) gives the following criteria for Attention-Deficit/Hyperactivity Disorder:

- Either (1) or (2) below:

1. six or more of the following symptoms of inattention have persisted for at least 6 months to a degree that is maladaptive and inconsistent with developmental level:

Inattention
- often fails to give close attention to details or makes careless mistakes in schoolwork, work, or other activities
- often has difficulty sustaining attention in tasks or play activities
- often does not seem to listen when spoken to directly
- often does not follow through on instructions and fails to finish schoolwork, chores, or work duties (not because of oppositional behavior or failure to understand instructions)
- often has difficulty organizing tasks and activities
- often avoids, dislikes, or is reluctant to engage in tasks that require sustained mental effort
- often loses things necessary for tasks or activities
- is often easily distracted by extraneous stimuli
- is often forgetful in daily activities

2. six or more of the following symptoms of hyperactivity- impulsivity have persisted for at least 6 months to a degree that is maladaptive and inconsistent with developmental level:

Hyperactivity
- often fidgets with hands or feet or squirms in seat
- often leaves seat in classroom or in other situations in which remaining seated is expected
- often runs about, climbs excessively or feels restless in situations where it is inappropriate
- often has difficulty playing or engaging in leisure activities quietly
- is often "on the go" or often acts as if "driven by a motor"

- often talks excessively

Impulsivity
- often blurts out answers before questions have been completed
- often has difficulty awaiting turn
- often interrupts or intrudes on others

Some hyperactive-impulsive or inattentive symptoms that caused impairment were present before the age of 7.

- Some impairment from the symptoms is present in two or more settings.
- There must be clear evidence of clinically significant impairment in social, academic, or occupational functioning.
- Symptoms do not occur exclusively during the course of a pervasive developmental disorder, schizophrenia, or other psychotic disorder, and are not better accounted for by another mental disorder.

Note that the criteria for inattention involve task-centered behavior, which is controlled by the executive functioning capacity of the frontal lobe. Criteria for hyperactivity/impulsivity relate to lack of inhibition, controlled by the motor activation capacity of the frontal lobe.

7
Major Brain Disorders, Part II

My mind is troubled, like a fountain stirred; and I myself see not the bottom of it.

William Shakespeare
Troilus and Cressida

Illness behavior interferes with personality behavior.
Robert A. Williams, M.D.

Chapter 7 will discuss those five brain disorders that are not typically associated with biological psychiatry. These types of brain dysfunction usually are associated with therapists (as seen with personality disorders), sleep specialists or neurologists. They include:

1. Personality disorders
2. Sleep disorders
3. Delirium
4. Dementia
5. Structural deficits, addiction and permanent metabolic deficits

Childhood brain disorders also are presented here.

Personality Disorders

Summary: Personality *traits* are enduring patterns of perception, relative to the environment and the self, that are exhibited in a broad range of social and personal contexts. When traits are inflexible and maladaptive, causing significant functional impairment, they are known as personality *disorders*.[1] Personality disorders usually become evident during adolescence or early adulthood.

In general, personality disorders are characterized by traits that result in maladaptive behavior. These traits, however, are greatly influenced by the content of an individual's life and, according to the situation, may be expressed adaptively or maladaptively.[2] Maladaptive traits include codependence, poor strategies of life, poor coping skills, and interpersonal stress. The recommended way to help individuals deal with these so-called "problems of life" is through therapy.

Antisocial Personality Disorder[3] (sociopathy) is in a category by itself because it is the only personality disorder that fits the medical model.[4] In this case related generators of behavior are *not* independent of the personality structure.[5] This disorder has a strong genetic determinant, usually presents before the age of 15, and is evident on a constant basis. In men, increased testosterone levels correlate with increased incidence of violent antisocial behavior. Sadly, there is no known treatment for sociopathy, and the only practical method that our society has found to deal with individuals who have this disorder is isolation, typically through incarceration.

Borderline Personality Disorder (BPD),[6] (one of the most commonly diagnosed personality disorders in mainstream psychiatry) is marked by a pervasive pattern of instability in interpersonal relationships, self-image, and affects as well as extreme impulsivity. It usually begins in early adulthood and is evident in a variety of situations. BPD, which is very difficult to treat,[7] has many of the same symptoms as a mood disorder, for which there are more treatment options. For this reason, BPD patients can greatly benefit from the same treatment that generally would be prescribed for mood disorder patients. Fig. 7-1 presents a comparison of BPD and mood disorder symptoms and depicts how BPD correlates with five criteria for major depression, four criteria for hypomania, and two criteria for mixed states. This leads to the conclusion that most borderline cases probably are caused by a form of affective disorder.

Consequences of an antisocial personality also can produce behavior that fits a borderline personality diagnosis. Fig. 7-2 shows the relationship of antisocial personality disorder criteria, consequences of antisocial personality disorder, and BPD criteria correlates.

At the Biological Psychiatry Institute we have had no problem rediagnosing patients who have been diagnosed originally with antisocial personality disorder, affective disorder (or a combination of these two disorders), BPD, or all these disorders.

Patients who present with an antisocial personality pattern are not well treated medically unless they have an associated mood disorder. (As mentioned previously, a medical treatment approach

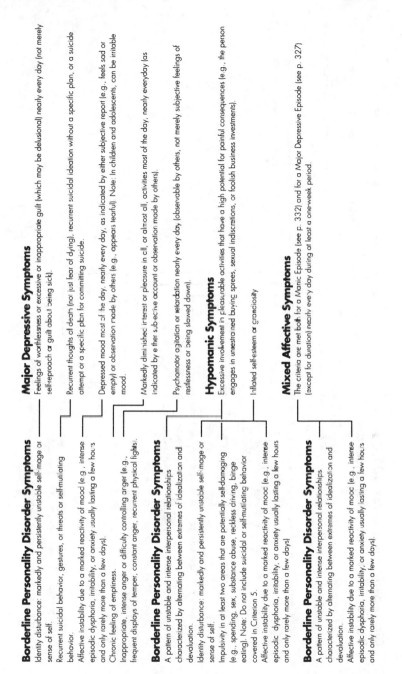

Figure 7-1. Symptoms/correlates of borderline personality disorder and mood disorder.

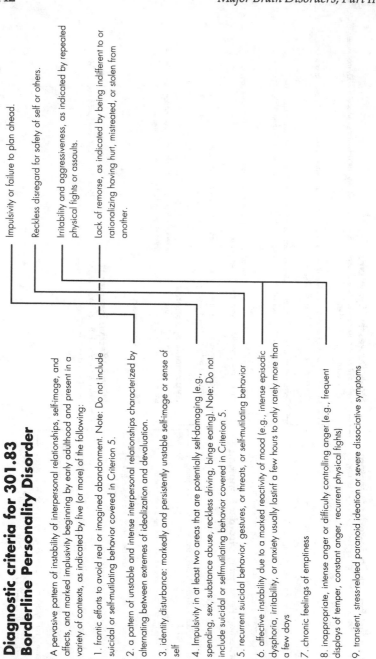

Figure 7-2. Symptoms/correlates of borderline personality disorder and antisocial personality disorder.

can be applied to mood disorder patients.) Instead of psychotherapy, however, programs that provide an extremely strong external structure (similar to the structure of prison) are most effective. Firm rules of engagement are required to avoid being manipulated by patients. For example, some BPD programs exclude *all* patients who use suicidal behavior for any purpose.[8]

Sleep Disorders

Summary: Sleep disorders prevent individuals from achieving adequate sleep and interfere with normal functioning. This type of brain disorder includes unusual behaviors during sleep (i.e., sleep walking or sleep terrors) that might endanger or disturb patients or others.

Sleep has three biological control mechanisms:

1. *Autonomic nervous system* [ANS] (suppression of sleep for survival)—Sympathetic arousal can cause cortical activation and inhibit sleep. An example of this would occur if an individual were very tired and about to fall asleep. Suddenly, he hears the sound of breaking glass somewhere in his house, is instantly wide awake and bolts to the phone to call "911."

2. *Homeostasis* (the amount of sleep needed)—When prolonged wakefulness produces a sleep debt (insufficient sleep), the brain produces a subjective assignment for sleepiness, which provides the motivation to reduce other human drives. In order to maintain homeostasis, the hypothalamus keeps track of the amount of sleep needed, the amount actually obtained, and alerts the awareness center when an individual has not had enough sleep.

3. *Circadian rhythm* (determination of the timing of sleep)—This pacemaker or timekeeper for regulating sleep is superimposed on the homeostatic effects of sustained wakefulness. The human circadian rhythm is reset daily by bright light, which maintains synchrony between environmental clocks (work/school) and the biological clock (sleep). Also, synchrony is maintained by the release of melatonin that promotes sleep at night (darkness facilitates the release of melatonin).

Normal sleep occurs when all three of the preceding biological control mechanisms work together to maximize opportunities for sleep.

1. The *autonomic nervous system* is involved with the following sleep hygiene (quieting the brain) issues:
   - quiet environment—sleeping environment is free of alerting mechanisms
   - increased muscle relaxation—physical tiredness often occurs progressively under natural conditions. Physical exercise at the time of sleep may have an activating affect but biofeedback can aid muscle relaxation.
   - decreased mental alertness—although mental relaxation occurs naturally, excessive anxiety and worry may delay sleep; meditation, hypnosis, and deep-breathing may hasten it. If an individual has developed conditioned mental alertness, stimulus control therapy (deconditioning) may help.
   - limited maladaptive associations—"foreign elements" that create an unnatural sleep environment should be minimized. For example, individuals who fall asleep watching television every night may not be able to go to sleep in bed. Similarly, infants or young children may only be able to sleep with a parent present. In both cases cognitive restructuring of sleep without television or a parent is achieved by slowly withdrawing such foreign elements from the sleep environment.

2. *Homeostasis* stimulates individuals to seek sufficient sleep during the normal sleep cycle, so that daytime naps can be avoided or limited.
3. *Circadian rhythm* stimulates the natural tendency to sleep and is governed by the biological clock in the hypothalamus; promotes the timing of sleep at night and wakefulness during the day.

When the autonomic nervous system, homeostasis, and circadian rhythm act together, natural sleep ensues. For instance, if an individual is relaxed because of calm thoughts, tired from the day's activities and is experiencing a rise in melatonin (which initiates circadian rhythm), sleep comes rapidly.

Let's look at the major disorders that can interfere with natural sleep:

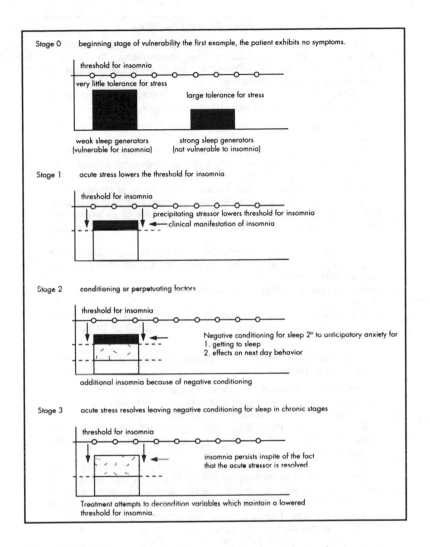

Stage 0   beginning stage of vulnerability the first example, the patient exhibits no symptoms.

threshold for insomnia

very little tolerance for stress

large tolerance for stress

weak sleep generators   strong sleep generators
(vulnerable for insomnia)   (not vulnerable to insomnia)

Stage 1   acute stress lowers the threshold for insomnia

threshold for insomnia

precipitating stressor lowers threshold for insomnia
clinical manifestation of insomnia

Stage 2   conditioning or perpetuating factors

threshold for insomnia

Negative conditioning for sleep 2° to anticipatory anxiety for
1. getting to sleep
2. effects on next day behavior

additional insomnia because of negative conditioning

Stage 3   acute stress resolves leaving negative conditioning for sleep in chronic stages

threshold for insomnia

insomnia persists inspite of the fact
that the acute stressor is resolved

Treatment attempts to decondition variables which maintain a lowered
threshold for insomnia.

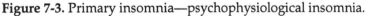

Figure 7-3. Primary insomnia—psychophysiological insomnia.

Primary Sleep Disorders are "primary" because they are related to an inherent problem in the sleep-regulating systems or they are not secondary to sleep disorders related to other mental disorders, general mental conditions or substance-induced sleep disorders.[9] Primary sleep disorders are classified as **dyssomnias** or **parasomnias**.

More About Primary Insomnia

Because primary insomnia is so common, it deserves special attention. A discussion about the mechanisms of psychophysiological insomnia follows, as well as a description of nonpharmacological treatments.

Primary insomnia is caused by a weak sleep generator of behavior. There are seven types of primary insomnia:

1. Psychophysiological Insomnia—caused by stress that provides negative conditioning for sleep.
2. Adjustment Sleep Disorder—caused by stress (conflict or environmental change), which results in emotional arousal (i.e., transient psychophysiological insomnia).
3. Sleep State Misperception—exists where there is complaint of insomnia in the absence of objective evidence of sleep disturbance. There is a weak link between sleep generators of behavior and subjective assignment, (or awareness), that one has had adequate sleep.
4. Sleep Onset Association Disorder—caused when association with an element (i.e., television) that distracts from sleep in the normal sleep environment.
5. Inadequate Sleep Hygiene—occurs in the presence of poor sleep habits.
6. Idiopathic Insomnia—insomnia that has been present since birth.
7. "Short Sleeper" Disorder—occurs when someone needs very little sleep.

There are two significant nonpharmacological techniques that can be used to facilitate sleep.

1. Relaxation techniques provide two functions for sleep:
   * decrease muscle tension that may prevent sleep
   * distract patient from anxiety about sleep

Examples of relaxation techniques include progressive relaxation, deep breathing (i.e., yoga), biofeedback, hypnosis, and cognitive relabeling.

2. Stimulus control attempts to "cancel" conditioning that undermines sleep by helping to reduce both primary and reactive factors involved with insomnia. The stimulus is the act of going to bed; the response is the inability to sleep because of increased anxiety at bedtime. The control is avoiding anxiety at bedtime.

Stimulus control guidelines include:
   * going to bed only when sleepy
   * using bed only for sleeping
   * establishing presleep routines

when unable to sleep, getting out of bed and engaging in nonstimulating activity
   * maintaining regular sleep schedule
   * avoiding day-time naps

In spite of good sleep hygiene, if a patient is unable to sleep, restricting time in bed can help consolidate sleep. Sleep restriction therapy may produce a gradual and steady decline in nocturnal wakefulness.

Dyssomnias, of which there are five major classifications, are caused by a disturbance in the amount, quality or timing of sleep and are characterized by excessive sleepiness or difficulty in initiating/ maintaining sleep.

1. *Primary insomnia* is due to a weak sleep generator (see "More About Primary Insomnia" on page 146 and Fig. 7-3).
2. *Primary hypersomnia* involves prolonged sleep episodes with daytime sleepiness or sleep. Apparently, in spite of sleep that appears normal, sleep is not restorative. Other notable behaviors include "sleep drunkenness" and autonomic behavior, such as not being aware of having driven to a particular place.
3. *Narcolepsy* involves the onset of sleep during awake periods. Presumably, sleep suppression mechanisms are defective, which causes the following essential features of narcolepsy:

   * Irresistible attacks of refreshing sleep
   * Cataplexy, or sudden loss of muscle tone
   * REM sleep during transition between sleep and wakefulness, which is manifested by hallucinations or sleep paralysis

4. *Breathing-related sleep disorders* disrupt normal sleep and cause daytime sleepiness.[10] Obstructive sleep apnea, which is accompanied by loss of spinal reflexes, is the most common breathing-related sleep disorder and is caused by paralysis or collapse of the upper airway in susceptible individuals. When the upper airway collapses, air flow may stop or be highly restricted. When oxygen levels drop, the patient is alerted and stops REM sleep. REM sleep deprivation may result in daytime somnolence.
5. *Circadian rhythm disorder* is a recurrent pattern of sleep disruption that results from a mismatch between an individual's endogenous circadian sleep-wake system and exogenous demands regarding the timing and duration of sleep.

A common subtype of circadian rhythm sleep disorder is delayed sleep phase syndrome [DSPS] ("night owl"). For example, an individual's sleep is delayed from 10 PM to 3 AM; if he or she is allowed to sleep late, there will be normal refreshing sleep. If he or she gets up early, there will be sleep deprivation and daytime somnolence. Normally, individuals have flexible circadian rhythms that adjust to morning light and nighttime darkness.

148 *Major Brain Disorders, Part II*

DSPS patients have fixed sleep patterns. Other circadian rhythm sleep disorders include jet lag and shift work.

Dyssomnias not otherwise specified include "restless leg syndrome" (idiopathic periodic limb movements or nocturnal myoclonus) and others.

Parasomnias are characterized by abnormal behavior or psychological events occurring during sleep or sleep-wake transition. This type of sleep disorder does not involve abnormalities of sleep mechanisms that initiate and maintain sleep or affect the timing of sleep. Parasomnias involve the activation of the autonomic system, motor system, or cognitive processes during sleep or sleep-wake transitions. Complaints involving parasomnias involve unusual behavior during sleep rather than insomnia or excessive daytime sleepiness. There are three common types of parasomnias.

1. *Nightmare disorder* (affects *cognitive function*) consists of repeated frightening dreams, arising from the REM sleep phase, that lead to awakenings. On awakening, dream content is remembered and patients are alert.
2. *Sleep terror disorder* (affects *autonomic function*) is comprised of repeated episodes of sleep terrors during which there is autonomic arousal and intense fear. It is difficult to awaken individuals, and they have no clear dream recall; in fact, the next day there usually is amnesia about the event. Sleep terror may occur during Stage 3 or 4 of sleep but most often during the first third of sleep and last 1 to 10 minutes. Episodes are usually accompanied by yelling, screaming, crying or incoherent vocalization.
3. *Sleep walking disorder* (affects *motor function*) consists of repeated episodes of complex motor behavior (such as, walking) during sleep. This disorder occurs during slow wave sleep (first third of sleep). During episodes, patients have reduced alertness and later reduced recall about the sleep walking event. After the episode, patients experience brief periods of confusion and then recover full alertness.

Delirium/Encephalopathy

Summary: Delirium/Encephalopathy,[11] which occurs secondary to metabolic (biochemical) effects on the brain, is an acute, diffuse, reversible process that involves inattention (frontal lobes), rambling speech (left tempoparietal area) and other brain problems. If metabolic processes cause permanent or structural changes in the brain, then the specific area of dysfunction is designated as a specific lobe dysfunction, i.e., frontal lobe syndrome.

Metabolic stress that causes reversible dysfunction is created by either adding an element that should not be present (i.e., carbon monoxide) or subtracting an element that should be present (i.e., oxygen). The process that causes delirium (reversible) can advance and produce permanent brain damage (irreversible).

In DSM-III-R disorders of this type were classified in a section entitled "Organic Mental Syndromes and Disorders." The term, "organic mental disorder," is no longer used in the DSM-IV because it implies that "nonorganic" mental disorders do not have a biological basis.[12] This modified definition is an example of how psychiatry is developing a greater understanding of brain disorders and is dispelling some of the myths that have surrounded this medical specialty for years.

Delirium[13] is characterized by a disturbance of consciousness and a change in cognition that develops over a brief period of time and involves dysfunction of the frontal lobes or other areas of the brain.[14] Causes of delirium are many and include:[15]

1. Sudden loss of nutrients required by the brain (i.e., sugar, vitamines/hormones, oxygen, etc.)
2. Traumatic events that affect brain metabolism (i.e., head trauma, seizures)
3. Toxins that affect brain metabolism (i.e., infections, heavy metals, insecticides)
4. Drugs that affect brain metabolism[16]
   • Direct effects
   • Withdrawal effects—Alcohol withdrawal can cause seizures and delirium tremors

Delirium may occur in mild forms and present as one problem related to a single generator of behavior or may occur in comparatively severe forms when several generators of behavior are involved. In the early stages of delirium, the most vulnerable generators of behavior will be affected first. The metabolic "cut" through the brain may affect only one generator of behavior. In the case of chronic obstructive lung disease, anxiety or depression commonly are seen in the early phases of the disease. As the illness progresses and delirium worsens, the metabolic cut through the brain grows deeper and more generators of behavior are affected. When the brain stem is involved, death may ensue.

The brain's metabolic reserve decreases with age. For example, a bladder infection in a young woman may cause irritability, whereas it might bring about delirium in an older woman. Stress in the emergency room may cause simple anxiety in a young person but extreme confusion (frontal lobe dysfunction) in someone who is elderly. Fatigue and sleep deprivation may cause irritability for a young person but acute psychotic agitation (the "sundown syndrome") in an elderly individual.

Dementia

Summary: Dementia is characterized by development of multiple cognitive[17] deficits, including memory impairment, that are caused by a general neurological condition, effects of a substance or the combined effects of multiple diseases. Because the generators of behavior for dementia are located in particular lobes of the brain, this disorder is said to involve specific lobe dysfunction.

The generator of behavior that is most sensitive to the dementing process is memory. Dementia can be primary (caused by hereditary factors or Alzheimer's disease)[18] or secondary (caused by stroke, HIV disease, head trauma, Parkinson's disease, or general medical conditions).

While age is a major risk factor for dementia, certain characteristics (i.e., minor forgetfulness, disinhibition, and language changes)[19] accompany the aging process and are not necessarily an indication of dementia. The diagnosis of dementia involves testing different lobes of the brain through use of one or more standardized exams. One of the most frequently used is the Mini Mental Status Exam (MMSE) on which a score of 20 or less typically correlates with dementia. Unfortunately, there is no decisive treatment for dementia.

As dementia progresses, patients remain alert and experience no decreased level of consciousness, although all lobes of the brain eventually may be involved. Because the brain loses its ability to maintain homeostasis, death generally occurs as a result of accidental falls, pneumonia, dehydration or infection.

A Biological View of Alcoholics Anonymous' 12-Step Program

Alcoholics Anonymous (AA) was born in May 1935 when Bill W. met Bob S. (a surgeon) and began the 3-year process of developing AA's 12-step program and the *Big Book* (Thompson R. *Bill W.* New York: Harper & Row; 1975:214). Prior to this effort, alcoholism was treated with traditional psychiatric treatment (i.e., analysis), which was notably unsuccessful. Over the next 15 years AA's 12 traditions were developed and later the organization's "Constitution" (the 12 concepts and 6 warranties) was formulated. The result of this lengthy development process was a program that provides the tools to cope with the stressors of life and is still our society's most effective method for maintaining sobriety (*Psychiatric Annals* 1992;22(1):410).

Today, AA's 12-Step program is the mainstay referral for the biological treatment of addiction. (Addiction disorders traditionally are referred to a biological psychiatrist for treatment.) Because of the high comorbidity of psychiatric illness (i.e., major depression, panic disorders, sleep disorders, eating disorders, social phobia, bipolar disorders, and many others), it has been found that "combining professional medical treatment with the AA program results in treatment improvements" (*Psychiatric Annals*).

The following biological view of AA's 12-Step program attempts to explain how each step fits into the neuropsychiatric model of biological psychiatry. The neuropsychiatric objective is to control illness behavior so that outward behavior reflects personality. The objective of sobriety is the absence of alcohol or intoxicant use, which is the same as control of illness behavior or craving. These objectives are identical.

Step 1 "We admitted we were powerless over alcohol—that our lives had become unmanageable."

In other words, medical disorders are *not* disorders of will or self-control ("powerless"). In fact, as the neuropsychiatric model shows, addictive generators of behavior are produced independent of the personality and interfere with normal capacity to function and manage life ("unmanageable").

Normally, behavior is regulated by frontal lobe executive function. It is a natural assumption that, if we *experience* behavior, we can *regulate* it. Addictive behavior, however, is generated independent of personality and frontal lobe executive function. When the addictive generator reaches a certain threshold, then an individual is "powerless" to control the thoughts or cravings. Step 1 explicitly states that addiction is a *medical disorder*.

Step 2 "Came to believe that a power greater than ourselves could restore us to sanity."

One of the neuropsychiatric principles states there are multiple determinants of behavior that fall within three primary categories—biological, psychosocial, and spiritual. In the 1930s Bill W., one of the AA cofounders, made a fundamental observation that there was overlap between spiritualism and the capacity to control the biological drive to drink. This observation is consistent with the concept of overlapping determinants of behavior.

The phrase, "restore us to sanity," meshes with the neuropsychiatric concepts of psychosis and brain dysfunction. Basically, addiction is produced by independent generators of

---

behavior, just as any other form of psychosis or neuropsychiatric disorder.

Step 3 "Made a decision to turn our will and our lives over to the care of God as we understood Him."

The neuropsychiatric model of the brain includes *awareness*. Different parts of the brain feed into frontal lobe awareness, providing an experience of different subjective assignments, from the five senses to the capacity to devise and execute a plan.

The phrase, "made a decision," strongly suggests that executive function can direct attention to spiritual awareness. The phrase, "to turn our will and our lives over to the care of God as we understand Him," is a statement that recognizes the spiritual capacity that is part of each person on earth. Step 3 states that executive function can be used to focus on spiritual capacities to help control alcoholic behavior.

Perhaps one reason that the spiritual focus works is that addictive input is on the opposite end of the array of subjective assignments from awareness. By maintaining a spiritual focus, addictive input can be avoided or disconnected (see "Temporary Disconnection Syndrome" in Chapter 6). When patients attempt to control addiction by focusing executive function on awareness of addiction or associated cravings, they are unsuccessful. If patients focus on spiritual awareness, the addiction generator temporarily disconnects from awareness and provides sobriety.

Step 4 "Made a searching and fearless moral inventory of ourselves."

Step 4 focuses on social determinants of behavior. Society teaches moral structure, which is contained in the frontal lobes. If individuals deviate from social mores (i.e., pursuing addiction), then guilt and, possibly, social rejection and isolation are experienced. The net effect of deviant behavior is stress. For the alcoholic the cascading stress effects of being labeled as an "alcoholic" are severe. Examination of behavior in relationship to social standards can provide a good approximation of the impact of social stressors contributing to illness behavior. Because social stress decreases the threshold for all illness and may bring out vulnerable generators of behavior, it makes sense to evaluate social determinants of behavior and to reduce stressful influences.

Step 5 "Admitted to God, to ourselves and to another human being the exact nature of our wrongs."

Alcohol or other addicting intoxicants diminish social values because the addicting substance and consequences of intoxication create a set of priorities of their own that tend to blur moral judgment. Step 5 reestablishes a heightened awareness of personal values (as related to personality) and encourages resolution of social conflict or stress (contributing to illness) by admitting and sharing mistakes ("wrongs"). Resolving social conflict tends to decrease the likelihood of illness.

Both steps 4 and 5 relate to social determinants within the brain (i.e., moral values).

Step 6 "Were entirely ready to have God remove all these defects of character."

A Biological View of Alcoholics Anonymous' 12-Step Program continued

Step 6 refers to psychological determinants of behavior. The neuropsychiatric model of the brain defines personality ("character") as the overlapping matrix of all generators of behavior in the brain. The phrase, "defects of character," refers to maladaptive generators of behavior, which can reduce the threshold for illness. The phrase, "we're entirely ready," means individuals are proactive in utilizing executive function to develop strategies for dealing with maladaptive behavior. "God" is used to symbolize honesty in trying to self-monitor behavior.

Step 7 "Humbly ask Him to remove our shortcomings."

Step 7 is the recognition that individuals must develop strategies that minimize the stress that results from maladaptive behavior. "Him" refers to the spiritual intuitiveness or motivation that logically follows when maladaptive behavior is defined. (Step 6 defines maladapative behavior, while Step 7 seeks to alleviate it.)

Step 8 "Made a list of all persons we had harmed, and became willing to make amends to them all."

The social system each individual inhabits has a major impact on mental health. Close friends and relatives comprise an essential support system. (AA meetings provide important social support systems that encourage sobriety.) When friends and relatives become alienated because of addictive behavior, addicts become socially isolated. Social isolation is extremely stressful and is even an acknowledged form of torture or punishment (i.e., solitary confinement). Step 8 recognizes the source of social isolation (i.e., "a list of all persons we had harmed") and the need to become motivated to do something about it (i.e., "become willing to make amends to them all").

Step 9 "Made desired amends to such people wherever possible, except when to do so would injure them or others."

Step 9 features several functions to help the addict.

1. Addictive behavior cannot be seen, but the consequences (i.e., harm to specific individuals) are manifest. Steps 8 and 9 help the addict focus on consequences so that belief about being an addict can be developed.

2. A sensitivity to the social consequences of addictive behavior is critical. Attempts to make amends will clearly show the irreversibility of many broken social relationships that result from addictive behavior (more consequences).

3. Attempts to make amends allow addicts to identify their true friends. Under the influence of intoxicants, the ability to discern character and choose healthy friends is compromised. As addiction becomes controlled, addicts can learn to find people in their environments who are forgiving, accepting, and supportive of addiction recovery.

4. Addicts will attempt to establish a supportive social environment and avoid social isolation.

Both Steps 8 and 9 relate to external social support systems.

Step 10 "Continued to take personal inventory and, when we were wrong, promptly admitted it."

In Step 10, "personal inventory" is the neuropsychiatric equivalent of awareness. When patients attempt to identify illness in the neuropsychiatric model, they learn to recognize certain symptoms or potential stressors. The following algorithm fits this concept of "personal inventory" or self-monitoring.

1. Onset of symptoms of illness (cravings)
With self-monitoring
- Attend AA meetings
- Call AA sponsor

If biologic comorbid condition exists
- Seek biological psychiatric help, as needed

Without self-monitoring
- Surrender to addictive cravings caused by unusual content of life (i.e., grief, PTSD, high stress, abuse)

2. Ongoing presence of unusual content of life
With self-monitoring
- Attend AA meetings
- See counselor, as needed

Without self-monitoring
- Display of maladaptive behavior

3. Manifestation of maladaptive behavior
With self-monitoring
- Follow 12-step program, attend AA meetings
- See counselor, as needed

Without self-monitoring
- Display of spiritual problems

4. Manifestation of spiritual problems
With self-monitoring
- Follow 12-step program, attend AA meetings, focus on spiritual choices or spiritual counseling

Without self-monitoring
- Return to Step 1

The phrase, "when we were wrong," describes maladaptive behavior that contributes to decreasing the threshold for illness. The phrase, "promptly admitted it," means that addicts cannot deny awareness of their own behavior that either represents illness or activity that reduces the threshold for illness.

Step 11 "Sought through prayer and meditation to improve our conscious contact with God as we understood Him, praying only for knowledge of His will for us and the power to carry that out."

Step 11 is a restatement of the need to maintain focus on spirituality. The basic element of all spirituality relates to acceptance of life and release of the obsessive burden to control. "Knowledge of His will" refers to acceptance of life, and "the power to carry that out" refers to the flow of life. "Meditation to improve our conscious contact with God" signifies the focus of executive function on spiritual awareness. Step 11 reiterates that spiritual focus temporarily disconnects the addictive generator of behavior and facilitates sobriety.

Step 12 "Having had a spiritual awakening as the result of these steps, we tried to carry this message to alcoholics and to practice these principles in all our affairs."

Step 12 provides two primary behavioral determinants for addicts:

A Biological View of Alcoholics Anonymous' 12-Step Program continued

1. "We tried to carry this message to alcoholics" provides a constant reminder to alcoholics that other individuals' addictive behavior is more easily recognized than one's own. Helping others provides a continuous input to addicts' awareness of the consequences of addictive behavior.

2. "To practice these principles in all our affairs" states that general application of healthy life principles tends to promote lifetime maintenance of these principles.

In summary, AA's 12-Step program fits the neuropsychiatric model of the brain:

1. Addiction is a medical disorder.

2. A focus on the consequences of illness is necessary in order to recognize illness.

3. A spiritual focus temporarily disconnects the addictive generator of behavior from awareness and provides a means to maintain sobriety.

4. Stressors that lower the threshold for illness must be addressed.

5. Addiction is a lifelong illness. It is necessary to continuously monitor for illness and variables that reduce the illness threshold.

Structural Defects (brain dysfunction secondary to changes in brain structure)

Summary: Structural disorders are caused either by direct physical contact (i.e., trauma, tumor, multiple sclerosis, aneurysm, stroke, arteriovenous malformation), or by direct toxic contact[20] (i.e., alcohol and drug addiction).

Structural abnormalities in the brain can be caused by a variety of elements:

1. Aneurysms
2. Arteriovenous malformations
3. Brain abscesses
4. Calcium deposits
5. Chemicals
6. Foreign bodies
7. Head trauma
8. Hydrocephalus
9. Parasites
10. Strokes

Any structural change in the brain, depending on its location, can cause the brain to fail in its usual capacities and result in a brain disorder. Investigation of a brain syndrome involves ruling out secondary causes of brain syndrome, such as structural lesions. Patient history (including drug use, family history, and patterns of illness) as well as physical and neurological exams are used to rule out structural lesions; lab tests are used to eliminate metabolic disorders that may cause brain dysfunction.

With regard to toxic contact, chemicals can have particularly widespread structural effects. For example, alcohol may cause shrinkage of the cerebellum, which can cause difficulty with gait and poor coordination of movements.[21] The most profound structural changes, however, are seen in the nucleus accumbens. Addiction, in fact, occurs when an addictive substance and the nucleus accumbens interact to form a permanent independent generator of behavior (i.e., a craving for a specific substance).

Addictive generators of behavior exist independent of personality and create obsessive thoughts about the intake of a substance not normally desired. Once structural change (the capacity to experience cravings for a substance) has occurred in the nucleus accumbens, it lasts a lifetime. For example, although an individual may have stopped smoking years ago, the thought of smoking a cigarette may reoccur. If an individual has never smoked a cigarette, the notion of smoking a cigarette will not usually come to mind. The same can be said for any other addictive substance, such as cocaine or alcohol.

The lifetime endurance of addiction is no different from the lifetime presence of other illnesses, such as anxiety disorders, manic depressive illness, or schizophrenia. The histories of patients who participate in Alcoholics Anonymous (AA) are full of references to regressing into addictive behavior, whether they have been "dry" for 5, 10, or 20 years. This is why AA patients are continually focused on "one day at a time" throughout their entire lives. (See "A Biological View of Alcoholics Anonymous' 12-Step Program" on pages 151–155.)

The brain's vulnerability to addictive substances is determined by several factors:

1. Genetic vulnerability of the brain
2. Amount of substance ingested and period of time over which it is ingested
3. Method by which a substance is ingested
4. Availability of substance

Drug and Alcohol Addiction: A Special Message for Young People

In this book, we have discussed many of the human brain's miraculous capacities. From a broad perspective, the brain has the capacity to reflect in countless ways the outside world and express awareness of elements in that world. It has the capacity for complex thought, robotics, and spiritualism. More specifically, the frontal lobes of the brain govern executive function or the capacity to focus awareness, to plan, and execute tasks. All individuals who possess normal brain capacity have the ability to control brain function through executive function or the "will."

Brain disorders are not disorders of "will" or self-control; rather, they produce behavior that is independent of individual personality. Addiction, like depression, anxiety, and obsessive compulsive disorder, is a brain disorder and occurs when the nucleus accumbens in the frontal lobes creates the desire for a substance (i.e., a cigarette or a can of beer) that is not normally ingested. (Read more about nicotine addiction in the May 1997 edition of *The Harvard Mental Health Letter*, volume 13, number 11, pages 1–4.) Addiction is present when the addiction generator of behavior, instead of the usual executive control, directs behavior.

What motivates individuals, especially young people, to begin smoking or taking drugs?

- positive sensations, including relaxation and dreamlike states
- attempts to gain independence, defiance of authority
- advertising
- social acceptance

Aside from the major health risks associated with drug and alcohol use, addictive substances *permanently* change the brain's basic structure. This is exemplified by the smoker who always will have the capacity to generate thoughts about wanting to smoke. (The previously cited issue of *The Harvard Mental Health Letter* states that in one study, 20 percent of former smokers expressed cravings to smoke 5 to 10 years after quitting smoking.) It is important to remember though that thoughts about cigarettes are not generated by a healthy brain but are produced by a brain disorder called addiction.

Making the conscious choice to use drugs or alcohol is a decision to give up control of the brain. It means being a slave to the addictive process itself. It also means being a victim of alcohol/cigarette company executives who seek to lead young people into lifelong addiction. "Say 'no' to drugs" (and alcohol) is more than an advertising slogan. It is a reminder to young people that *they* have the right to choose the course of their own lives and not to abdicate that right to a foreign substance.

All illnesses, including those of the addictive type, follow a particular course. Tobacco, alcohol, and other substances, for example, may be used adaptively at first. Preadolescents and adolescents, whose brains are still developing, are especially vulnerable to cultural forces. For individuals in these age groups, social pressure to smoke cigarettes is very high, and tobacco companies have made the most of this situation; more than 90 percent of those who are addicted to cigarettes are "hooked" by the age of 18.[22] (See "Drug and Alcohol Addiction: A Special Message for Young People" on page 157.)[23]

As the sedative and euphoric effects of tobacco and alcohol are discovered, they begin to be used as ways to cope with stress. Individuals appreciate the calmness and greater sense of well-being they feel when they are smoking or drinking. Many fail to recognize that their addiction is intensifying and they are gradually losing control of their ability *not* to use foreign substances. (Remember, addiction is not simply a disorder of will or self-control; it is a disease.)[24] The motivation for drinking and smoking transitions from social and psychological reasons to physical reasons. As adaptive behavior decreases, the more DSM-IV criteria for substance abuse are reflected.[25]

Finally, addicted individuals experience anxiety, depression and other symptoms of illness, either as direct toxic effects of substance abuse or as withdrawal effects. The ongoing use of tobacco, alcohol, and other substances temporarily alleviates symptoms of withdrawal and masks the disease process by satisfying the cravings. Ultimately, addiction can pave the way for severe depression, anxiety disorders, and suicide.

When individuals *do* seek treatment and overcome their addiction, some ask, "Can I ever drink again?" or, "Can I ever smoke again?"—questions that make most former addicts who have undergone treatment shudder because they know the answer in both cases is, "No." The question that should be asked is not "Can I ever drink or smoke again?" but "*Why* can't I ever drink or smoke again?" Unfortunately, addiction is a poorly understood and inadequately researched area of medicine. The answers to most questions about addiction are based on anecdotal studies, not scientific facts. In many instances, the AA philosophy toward controlling addiction circumvents most questions by relying on the day-by-day approach to sobriety. Fortunately, for many, the AA philosophy works.[26]

Childhood Disorders

The principles of child psychiatry are the same as those previously presented with regard to adult psychiatry. In fact, pervasive developmental disorders of childhood exemplify many principles of brain basics and are characterized by severe and progressive impairment in many areas of development.

Pervasive[27] Developmental Disorders (PDDs) affect several lobes of the brain and types of function:[28]

• reciprocal social interaction	social part of brain (frontal lobe)
• communication skills	language generator (left temporoparietal)
• stereotyped behavior	obsessive compulsive generator (basal ganglia)
• interests and activities generators	frontal lobe

"The qualitative impairments that define these conditions are distinctly deviant relative to the individual's developmental or mental age."[29] This statement means that in terms of brain basics:

1. The brain follows a genetic timeline in terms of development of normal brain function.
2. If, at a given time, expected brain development fails, "impairment" or brain failure is seen.

It should be noted that PDDs include cognitive disorders (i.e., mental retardation). The prognosis, or measurement of how well a patient will do over time, corresponds with the level of mental retardation. The prognosis worsens as the level of retardation increases. The PDDs are:

1. Autistic Disorder
2. Rett's Disorder
3. Childhood Disintegrative Disorder (CDD)
4. Asperger's Disorder
5. Pervasive Disorder (not otherwise specified)

Autistic Disorder[30] is typified by early onset (less than 3 years of age), diffusive brain dysfunction that affects social interaction, language, and play (i.e., usual early childhood activities). Associated clinical findings include mental retardation and any other possible brain dysfunction. Common associated behaviors (and the brain region that is affected) include:

1. ADD symptoms (basal ganglia)

2. Impulse disorder (frontal lobes)
   • temper tantrums
   • self-injury
3. Eating disorder (hypothalamus)
4. Sensory dysfunction (thalamus)
   • high threshhold for pain
   • audio oversensitivity
5. Sleep disturbance (hypothalamus)
6. Mood disorder (limbic system)
7. Phobias (brain stem)

Autistic disorder may be primary or secondary to "encephalitis, phenylketonuria, tuberous sclerosis, Fragile X Syndrome, anoxia [absence of oxygen] during birth or maternal rubella."[31]

Rett's Disorder[32] is the development of multiple specific deficits following a period of normal functioning after birth. This particular disorder only affects females. Following birth, genes follow a complicated path that dictates the development of the brain. Any problem along the genetic timeline can cause brain dysfunction.

Between 5 and 48 months of age children with Rett's Disorder develop brain dysfunction that is progressive, as opposed to autistic children whose brain dysfunction is present from the time of birth. Rett's children *become* symptomatic, although the clinical symptoms are similar to those seen in autistic children.

Childhood Disintegrative Disorder (CDD)[33] is marked by regression in multiple areas of functioning, following at least 2 years of apparently normal development. Symptoms of this disorder are similar to those seen in autistic and Rett's children, but in CDD the onset is later and both males and females may be affected. Between 2 and 10 years of age children experience progressive and diffuse brain failure. This disorder is associated with severe mental retardation and a high incident of seizure disorder.

Asperger's Disorder[34] is characterized by severe and sustained impairment of social interaction and the development of restricted patterns of behavior, interests, and activities.

Basically, Asperger's Disorder affects the social part of the frontal lobes and is associated with features of OCD. Asperger's does not involve language or cognition, but socially inappropriate language always is present. Mild forms of Asperger's Disorder may involve social functioning without OCD.

Summary (Chapters 6 and 7)

The 10 major classifications of brain disorders and five types of childhood disorders are diagnosed according to the 10-step process described in Chapter 1. Each type of disorder represents a dysfunction in a particular region of the brain, some of which evolved for adaptive purposes. One of the most significant ways to identify brain dysfunction is through the clusters of signs and symptoms described in the DSM-IV.

Identification of a specific brain dysfunction does not define illness. Whether the brain fails in its usual capacities because of genetics or as a result of the presence of one or more other illnesses, the precise cause of failure is not reflected in the clinical presentation of failure. The brain fails in its usual capacities with predictable clusters of signs and symptoms regardless of the cause.

The first step in helping someone who has a neuropsychiatric disorder is to *recognize* brain failure. It is the responsibility of the neuropsychiatrist to *define* the illness, based on age of onset, course of illness, response to medications, family history, physical examination, and lab tests. The purpose of chapters 6 and 7 is to provide DSM-IV behavioral clusters and brief descriptions of illnesses to enhance the reader's capacity to identify brain failure.

References

1. The DSM-IV (p. 633) gives the following criteria for Personality Disorder:

    - An enduring pattern of inner experience and behavior that deviates from the expectations of the individual's culture in two or more of the following areas: (a) ways of perceiving and interpreting self, other people, and events, (b) the range, intensity, ability, and appropriateness of emotional response, (c) interpersonal functioning, and (4) impulse control.
    - The enduring pattern is inflexible and pervasive across a broad range of personal and social siutations.
    - The enduring pattern leads to clinically significant distress in important areas of functioning.
    - The pattern is stable and of long duration with an onset that can be traced back at least to adolescence or early adulthood.
    - The enduring pattern is not better accounted for as a manifestation or consequence of another mental disorder.

- The enduring pattern is not due to the direct physiologic effects of a substance or a general medical condition.

2. For example, the trait of obsessiveness can be adaptive in the workplace when applied to computer programming tasks but maladaptive when applied to interpersonal relationships.
3. The DSM-IV (pp. 649–650) gives the following criteria for Antisocial Personality Disorder:
   - There is a pervasive pattern of disregard for and violation of the rights of others, occurring since age 15, as indicated by three of more of the following:

     1. failure to conform to social norms with respect to lawful behaviors
     2. deceitfulness, as indicated by repeated lying, use of aliases or conning others for personal gain
     3. impulsiveness or failure to plan ahead
     4. irritability and aggressiveness
     5. reckless disregard for safety of self or others
     6. consistent irresponsibility
     7. lack of remorse

   - The individual is at least 18 years of age.
   - There is evidence of Conduct Disorder before the age of 15.
   - The occurrence of antisocial behavior is not exclusively during schizophrenic or manic episodes.

4. This is the only personality disorder that is formally diagnosed at the Biological Psychiatry Institute.
5. With personality disorders, behavior that occurs within the physiology of the personality structure is subject to will and self-control. Therapy is designed to minimize or redirect behavior to gain a higher level of adaptability.
6. The DSM-IV (p. 654) gives the following criteria for Borderline Personality Disorder:

   - A pervasive pattern of instability of interpersonal relationships, self-image, marked impulsivity that begins in early adulthood and at least five of the following traits:

     1. frantic efforts to avoid real or imagined abandonment
     2. pattern of unstable and intense interpersonal relationships that alternates between extremes of idealization and devaluation
     3. persistently unstable sense of self

4. impulsivity in at least two self-damaging areas, i.e., spending, sex, substance abuse, reckless driving, binge eating
5. recurrent suicidal behavior or self-mutilating behavior
6. affective instability due to marked mood reactivity
7. chronic feeling of emptiness
8. inappropriate, intense anger or difficulty controlling anger
9. stress-related paranoid ideation or severe disassociative symptoms

7. At the Biological Psychiatry Institute, no patient ever receives the diagnosis of "borderline personality disorder."
8. My advice to individuals who are involved with those who have been diagnosed as antisocial personalities is to put as much distance as possible between themselves and those with this particular type of disorder.
9. Insomnia or hypersomnia is a sleep disturbance causally related to another mental disorder (delirium as a cause of insomnia is excluded). Additional diagnosis of insomnia or hypersomnia is made only when the sleep disturbance is the dominant complaint and severe enough to warrant independent clinical attention, as illustrated in the following examples:

Mental Disorder	*Sleep Disturbance*
Major depression	Difficulty falling asleep; early morning wakening
Bipolar disorder	Hypersomnia
Panic disorder	Wakening with panic
Generalized anxiety disorder	Difficulty falling asleep
Schizophrenia	Wandering at night; reversal of circadian rhythm; trouble falling asleep, maintaining sleep

Other disorders that are associated with sleep disturbances are adjustment disorder, somatoform disorders, and personality disorders.

Individuals with insomnia related to another mental illness may demonstrate the same conditional arousal and negative conditioning that individuals with primary insomnia demonstrate. From 40 to 60 percent of all hospital outpatients and up to 90 percent of patients with major depressive episodes have insomnia. From 35 to 50 percent of individuals presenting to sleep disorder centers have chronic insomnia.

Substance-induced sleep disorder occurs as a result of the direct physiological effects of a substance. This category also includes withdrawal effects from alcohol, amphetamines, cocaine, opiates, sedatives, hypnotics, and anxiolytics.

10. I believe breathing-related sleep disorders are primary sleep disorders because obstructive sleep apnea is secondary to sleep mechanisms, i.e., paralysis during REM sleep. The following breathing-related sleep disorders should be classified as secondary sleep disorders:

   - *Central Sleep Apnea Syndrome* is characterized by episodic cessation of ventilation during sleep, without airway obstruction. This disorder occurs more commonly in elderly patients, secondary to cardiac or neurological conditions that affect ventilatory regulation.
   - *Central Alveolar Hypoventilation Syndrome* is characterized by impaired ventilatory control, which is aggravated by sleep. In patients who are very overweight, lung oxygenation is inhibited (Pickwickian syndrome).

11. Depending on the initial complaint, other terms are used synonymously with "delirium," such as "encephalopathy" and "acute confusional state."
12. DSM-IV: 123.
13. DSM-IV (p. 129) gives the following criteria for Delirium:

   - Disturbance of consciousness with reduced ability to focus, sustain, or shift attention
   - A change in cognition or the development of a perceptual disturbance that is not better accounted for by a preexisting dementia
   - Disturbance develops over a short period of time and fluctuates during the day
   - There is evidence that the disturbance is caused by direct physiological consequences of a general medical condition

14. Note that the frontal lobes of the brain are the most advanced and also are the most sensitive to metabolic derangements. The frontal lobes *always* are the first part of the brain to be involved in delirium.
15. Conn DK. Delirium and other organic mental disorders. In: Sadavoy J, Lazarus L, Jarvik L, eds. *Comprehensive Review of Geriatric Psychiatry.* Washington, DC: American Psychiatric Press, Inc.; 1991:316.
16. Conn, 316.
17. "Cognitive" refers to the ability to perform specific tasks. These tasks include memory, language, abstract thinking, left-right orientation, executive planning, finger and facial recognition, skilled motor tasks, ability to dress, sensory recognition, ability to concentrate, and others.
18. DSM-IV (p. 142) gives the following criteria for Dementia of the Alzheimer's Type:

   - Development of multiple cognitive deficits manifested by both:

1. memory impairment
2. one or more of the following disturbances:
- language disturbance
- impaired ability to carry out motor activities
- failure to recognize or identify objects
- disturbance in executive functioning

Previously listed cognitive deficits can cause significant impairment in social or occupational functioning.

- Course is characterized by gradual onset and continuing cognitive decline
- Cognitive deficits listed in A1 and A2 are not due to any of the following:

  1. other central nervous system conditions, such as cerebrovascular disease, Parkinson's disease, Huntington's disease, subdural hematoma, hydrocephalus, and brain tumor
  2. systemic conditions that are known to cause dementia (i.e., hypothyroidism, vitamin B12 or folic acid deficiency, niacin deficiency, hypercalcemia, neurosyphilis, HIV infection)
  3. substance-induced conditions

- The deficits do not occur exclusively during the course of a delirium
- The disturbance is not better accounted for by another Axis I disorder (i.e., Major Depressive Disorder, Schizophrenia)

19. Older patients tend to be circumstantial and may include information that is not necessary for the answer to a given question.
20. DSM-IV (pp. 182–183) gives the following criteria for Substance Abuse:

  - A maladaptive pattern of substance use leading to clinically significant impairment or distress, as manifested by one or more of the following within a 12-month period:

    1. recurrent substance use resulting in a failure to fulfill major obligations at work, school or home
    2. recurrent substance use in physically hazardous situations
    3. recurrent substance-related legal problems
    4. continued substance use despite having persistent or recurrent social or interpersonal problems caused or exacerbated by the effects of the substance

- The symptoms have never met the criteria for substance dependence for this class of substance

21. Following is a list of alcohol's effects on certain regions of the brain:

• Nucleus accumbens	Addiction
• Cerebellum	Gait problems
• Entire brain	Alcoholic coma; withdrawal delirium
• Overactivation of brain	Withdrawal seizure
• Temporal lobes	Alcoholic hallucinosis (auditory hallucinations)
• High cortical functioning	Alcoholic dementia anxiety and agitation
• Brain stem	Large pupils/double vision

22. Preparing young people to prevent addictive illness or to deal with existing addiction is a vital social function. Today's strong social emphasis on avoidance of drugs and alcohol is a step in the right direction but, because addiction is a medical disorder of the brain, simultaneous emphasis on the neuropsychiatric brain model would provide a comprehensive explanation for the nature of addiction. For this reason, I recommend that AA's 12-step program and explanation of the neuropsychiatric brain model be part of a required course for students in 6th grade and beyond.

23. Nicotine Dependence: Part I. *The Harvard Mental Health Letter*, 1997;13(11):1–4.

24. As a medical disorder, addiction has several unique features:

- In general, it is not viewed by members of our society as being "medical." Remember, perceiving is *not* the same as believing.
- Lack of belief in the relationship between addiction and medical issues is reflected in the social stigma of alcoholism and other addictive disorders.
- Addictive generators of behavior bypass awareness and make it impossible for addicts to "see" their illness.
- The main form of treatment for addiction is nonmedical, i.e., Alcoholics Anonymous.

25. Unfortunately, medical technology has no provision for direct measurement of structural addictive changes in the brain. We only can observe the consequences of addiction and infer that addiction is present.

26. The "promises" that AA offers to its participants relate to the consequences of illness, since addicts cannot "see" their illness. The first phase of AA treatment involves evaluating the negative consequences of alcohol use, i.e., listing and making amends (when

appropriate) to individuals who have been harmed by the alcoholic. After patients have followed the AA program, they are directed to the positive consequences of sobriety as related in the AA "promises."

27. The term, "pervasive," is applied to this classification of childhood disorders because the frontal lobes, deep frontal lobes (basal ganglia), and left temporoparietal lobes are involved.

28. DSM-IV:65.

29. DSM-IV:65.

30. DSM-IV (pp. 70–71) gives the following criteria for Autistic Disorder:

- Symptoms must include a total of six or more items from sections 1, 2, and 3, at least two from section 1 and one each from sections 2 and 3:

    1. qualitative impairment in social interaction, as manifested by at least two of the following:
    - marked impairment in the use of multiple nonverbal behaviors, such as eye-to-eye gaze, facial expression, body postures and gestures to regulate social interaction
    - failure to develop peer relationships appropriate to developmental level
    - a lack of spontaneous seeking to share enjoyment, interests or achievements with other people (i.e., by a lack of showing, bringing, or pointing out objects of interest)
    - lack of social or emotional reciprocity

    2. qualitative impairments in communication as manifested by at least one of the following:
    - delay in, or total lack of, the development of spoken language (not accompanied by an attempt to compensate through alternative modes of communication, such as gesture or mime)
    - in individuals with adequate speech, marked impairment in the ability to initiate or sustain a conversation with others
    - stereotyped and repetitive use of language or idiosyncratic language
    - lack of varied, spontaneous make-believe play or social imitative play appropriate to developmental level

    3. restricted repetitive and stereotyped patterns of behavior, interests, and activities, as manifested by at least one of the following:
    - encompassing preoccupation with one or more stereotyped and restricted patterns of interest that is abnormal either in intensity of focus

- apparently inflexible adherence to specific, nonfunctional routines or rituals
- stereotyped and repetitive motor mannerisms (i.e., hand or finger flapping or twisting, or complex whole-body movements)
- persistent preoccupation with parts of objects

4. delays or abnormal functioning in at least one of the following areas, with onset prior to 3 years of age: (a) social interaction, (b) language as used in social communication, or (c) symbolic or imaginative play.

- the disturbance is not better accounted for by Rett's Disorder or Childhood Disintegrative Disorder.

31. DSM-IV:68.
32. DSM-IV (pp. 72–73) gives the following criteria for Rett's Disorder:

- All of the following:

   1. apparently normal prenatal and perinatal development
   2. apparently normal psychomotor development through the first 5 months after birth
   3. normal head circumference at birth

- Onset of all of the following after the period of normal development:

   1. deceleration of head growth between ages 5 and 48 months
   2. loss of previously acquired purposeful hand skills between ages 5 and 30 months with the subsequent development of stereotyped hand movements (i.e., hand-wringing or hand-washing)
   3. loss of social engagement early in the course (although often social interaction develops later)
   4. appearance of poorly coordinated gait or trunk movements
   5. severely impaired expressive and receptive language development with severe psychomotor retardation

33. DSM-IV (pp. 74–75) gives the following criteria for Childhood Disintegrative Disorder:

- Apparently normal development for at least the first two years after birth as manifested by the presence of age-appropriate verbal and nonverbal communication, social relationships, play, and adaptive behavior.

- Clinically significant loss of previously acquired skills (before age 10) in at least two of the following areas:
  1. expressive or receptive language
  2. social skills or adaptive behavior
  3. bowel or bladder control
  4. play
  5. motor skills

- Abnormalities of functioning in at least two of the following areas:
  1. qualitative impairment in social interaction (i.e., impairment in nonverbal behaviors, failure to develop peer relationships, lack of social or emotional reciprocity)
  2. qualitative impairments in communication (i.e., delay or lack of spoken language, inability to initiate or sustain a conversation, stereotyped and repetitive use of language, lack of varied make-believe play)
  3. restricted, repetitive and stereotyped patterns of behavior, interests and activities, including motor stereotypes and mannerisms

- The disturbance is not better accounted for by another specific pervasive developmental disorder or by schizophrenia

34. DSM-IV (p. 77) gives the following criteria for Asperger's Disorder:

- Qualitative impairment in social interaction, as manifested by at least two of the following:

  1. marked impairment in the use of multiple nonverbal behaviors, such as eye-to-eye gaze, facial expression, body postures and gestures to regulate social interaction
  2. failure to develop peer relationships appropriate to developmental level
  3. a lack of spontaneous seeking to share enjoyment, interests or achievements with other people (i.e., by a lack of showing, bringing or pointing out objects of interest to other people)
  4. lack of social or emotional reciprocity

- Restricted repetitive and stereotyped patterns of behavior, interests, and activities, as manifested by at least one of the following:

  1. encompassing preoccupation with one or more stereotyped and restricted patterns of interest that is abnormal either in intensity or focus
  2. apparently inflexible adherence to specific, nonfunctional routines or rituals

   3. stereotyped and repetitive motor mannerisms (i.e., hand or
      finger flapping or twisting, or complex whole-body
      movements)
   4. persistent preoccupation with parts of objects

- The disturbance causes clinically significant impairment in social,
  occupational, or other important areas of functioning.
- There is no clinically significant general delay in language (i.e.,
  single words used by age 2 years, communicative phrases used
  by age 3 years).
- There is no clinically significant delay in cognitive development
  or in the development of age-appropriate self-help skills,
  adaptive behavior (other than in social interaction), and curiosity
  about the environment in childhood.
- Criteria are not met for another specific pervasive developmental
  disorder or schizophrenia.

8
Psychiatric Diagnosis Based on the Open Model

The Brain—is wider than the Sky—
For—put them side by side—
The one the other will contain
With ease—and You—beside.

Emily Dickinson
Poem No. 632

The brain is the organ system of existence.

Robert A. Williams, M.D.

The open model is an all-inclusive model that includes the medical model, psychological theories and spirituality. Psychiatric diagnosis that stems from the open model seeks two objectives:

- to discern the presence of illness or disease in the brain (created either genetically and/or through acquired means) and to establish biological stability, the foundation for all behavior, through use of the medical model.
- to establish the presence of other determinants of behavior (i.e., psychosocial and spiritual determinants) following the determination of biological stability.

In the past, psychiatric illness has been very loosely defined in theoretical, instead of scientific, terms. Currently, psychiatry is in transition from an older nonscientific method of diagnosis to a scientific database created by the National Institute of Health (NIH) and other research organizations. The medical model, a scientific and rational approach to psychiatry, is the diagnostic technique used by the NIH.

The Diagnostic Process

Diagnosis according to the medical model is an evolutionary process. The first phase is descriptive and establishes the presence of biological illness. The second phase involves examination of laboratory values that relate to illness. Next comes assessment of abnormalities that relate to mechanisms of illness. The search for causes of illness through genetic analysis, family history and environmental influences is last.[1] Fig. 8-1 illustrates the evolutionary process of diagnosis for two sample disorders.

Unfortunately, laboratory tests for psychiatric illness are very weak, and tests for mechanisms of psychiatric illness are nonexistent. DNA testing is in the research phase and is not available for clinical use. There *are*, however, assessment tools designed to rule out medical illness that may secondarily cause psychiatric syndromes. For example, a thyroid profile may be used to rule out depression secondary to hypothyroidism.

As research uncovers more mechanisms of illness and more precisely defines genetic causes of illness, psychiatric diagnosis will become a more exact science. Currently, psychiatry emphasizes evaluation of the descriptive phase through identification of a specific collection of symptoms for each disorder, as described in the *Diagnostic and Statistical Manual of Mental Disorders* (DSM-IV).[2] Although each disorder is associated with a particular set of diagnostic criteria, multiple diagnoses are permitted and each general classification has a category called "not otherwise specified" for patients who have atypical symptoms. Some disorders have subtypes and/or degrees of severity (i.e., mild, moderate, in remission). Provisional (tentative) diagnoses can be made, as can differential diagnoses, which are based on insufficient data.[3]

A differential diagnosis consists of a list of all possible diagnoses. The most likely diagnosis usually is at the top of the list, with the least likely named last. For example, the differential diagnosis for a patient experiencing auditory hallucinations might include the following:

1. Psychotic depressions
2. Schizophrenia
3. Drug-induced psychosis
4. Manic psychosis
5. Delirium

Diagnostic Phases

Sample Diagnosis:
Major Depression

Sample Diagnosis:
Hypothyroidism

Descriptive Phase

- DSM-IV criteria for major depression
- Age of onset
- Cyclical course
- Response to medications
- Mental Status Exam

- Myxedema (puffy appearance)
- Increased sensitivity
- Dry skin
- Hair loss

Analysis of Abnormal Lab Values

- DST early escape
- Early REM sleep on sleep study

- Low thyroid levels in the blood

Analysis of Abnormalities Relating to Mechanisms of Illness

- Receptors

- Thyroid antibodies that decrease thyroid hormone output

Genetic/Environmental Analysis

- Genetic analysis
- Family history

- Genetic analysis
- Family history
- Environment

Figure 8-1. Evaluation of a medical diagnosis.

Another example is the schoolgirl who is extremely distracted in the classroom. Her differential diagnosis may include:

1. Attention deficit disorder
2. Panic disorder
3. Schizophrenia
4. Depression
5. Content-of-life elements, i.e., abuse, PTSD, high anxiety secondary to stress, grief

Clinical examples seen in Appendices L and M provide more detailed illustrations of differential diagnoses.

DSM-IV also provides a multiaxial system of classification as an amplification of the formerly described method of operational classification. Patients can be described in terms of each of the following five axes, although the first three are the only ones required for a formal diagnosis:[4]

Axis I	Primary psychiatric diagnosis
Axis II	Personality disorders that may or may not relate to the illness (since I do not recognize personality disorders—except for sociopathy—this axis is not utilized at the Biological Psychiatry Institute)
Axis III	Medical disorders that cause or contribute to Axis I
Axis IV	Psychosocial and environmental problems (i.e., stressors that reduce the threshold for illness)
Axis V	Global assessment of functioning (GAF)[5]

For example, a multiaxial evaluation for a patient whose chief complaint is "depression" might read as follows:

Axis I	Major depressive disorder, single episode, severe without psychotic features
Axis II	None
Axis III	None
Axis IV	On medical leave from job
Axis V	GAF = 50 (measured according to scale in DSM-IV)

The Williams Brain Model and associated principles generate information that is compatible with the multiaxial system. Specifically, the brain model demonstrates the amount of interference caused by an independent generator of behavior.

Causes of Illness Behavior

Any brain problem that disrupts function in one or more areas of life—self, interpersonal, social or industrial—is referred to as *illness*. Because most patients do not consult physicians unless they have problems, those seeking help for behavioral problems potentially have an illness, if brain dysfunction relates to behavioral problems.

When evaluating the *chief complaint* (a patient's problem, in his or her own words), it is important to look at the source of the behavior, whether it is biological, psychosocial, or spiritual. Consequences of biological illnesses potentially affect the form (manifestation) of all behavior. The chief complaint can be the result of:

1. symptoms of illness
2. psychological responses to illness
3. dynamic consequences of illness

Examples of psychological responses to illness behavior include:

Illness Behavior	Psychological Responses	Dynamic Consequences
Anxiety attacks	Fear of leaving home (Agoraphobia)	Social isolation, dependence (see Appendix N on panic attacks)
Hypomania	Anger	Marital discord
Obsessive Compulsive disorder (OCD)	Codependence	Interpersonal tension
Depression	Learned hopelessness, demoralization	Avoidance of intimacy

Behavioral problems can be caused by abnormal content (issues, situations, motivating factors) of life in the setting of normal brain function.[6] Psychological and dynamic problems can look the same as those caused by psychological and dynamic *consequences* of biological problems. Examples of psychological responses to content of life include:

Normal brain Abnormal Life Content	Psychological Responses	Dynamic Consequences
Threats to life, horror	PTSD	Social isolation
Major losses	Grief	Interpersonal stress
High stress	Anxiety, drug use	Decreased intimacy
Abuse	Formation of maladaptive "core beliefs"	Depression

The postwar experience of many Vietnam veterans exemplifies Posttraumatic Stress Disorder (PTSD). Lasting approximately 10 years, the Vietnam War affected the United States in many adverse ways; during that period in our history, the social sentiment was very antiwar and there was little popular support for the conflict itself, for the politicians and bureaucrats who funded it and for the men and women who fought overseas.

After having survived the combat horrors of Vietnam, veterans returned to the United States and experienced a host of negative consequences, such as social isolation, divorce, drug abuse, and unemployment. These and other factors caused severe emotional stress and led to PTSD for many veterans. The Veterans Administration has tried to mitigate the widespread PTSD problem with veteran support groups and programs offering intensive inpatient therapy, drug rehabilitation and special medical treatment.

Behavioral problems can occur in the setting of a normal brain with normal content of life but in the presence of poor "tools" for life. Maladaptive behavior in the setting of normal brain function is called neurosis. The consequences of neurotic behavior can look the same as those caused by biological sources:

Normal brain *Normal Life* *Content* (Neurosis)	*Psychological Responses*	*Dynamic Consequences*
Poor life strategies	Codependence, stress Demoralization	Interpersonal stress, relationship avoidance
Poor coping skills	Anxiety	Anxious relationships (see Appendix O on alcoholism)
Poor communication skills	Codependence, resentment of partner	Marital discord
Strong personality traits, i.e., histrionic	Emotional overreactivity	Marital arguments
narcissistic	Self-entitlement	Decreased intimacy

The case study of a young man who was seen at the Biological Psychiatry Institute illustrates how the consequences of neurotic behavior can have the appearance of biologically based consequences.

A 20-year-old white male of low-average intelligence had problems with finances in that he impulsively spent money on items he did not need. So-called friends took advantage of him. The patient had a high school education but was in special education classes and had a job at a restaurant bussing dishes. He was highly dependent on his parents to rescue him from his financial problems, including his rent payments. He had no history of psychiatric treatment and no family history of psychiatric disorders. He smoked cigarettes but used no other drugs. His medical work-up was negative.

The patient's exam revealed a calm young man who spoke in a naive fashion. Mood was euthymic. Affect was full-range. Motor level was normal. No psychosis was present. Cognition was slow, although the patient scored 25 out of 30 points on the Mini Mental Status Exam.

The patient did not satisfy the DSM-IV criteria for illness. The content of his life was not severe. He exhibited poor financial strategies of life with codependence on his family and high financial stress; he was referred to a counselor to develop appropriate financial strategies. Specifically, the patient's monthly earnings were budgeted and he was given a daily allotment to spend. This plan worked and the patient's codependence and stress decreased.

Following are self-imposed behaviors with biological consequences:

Normal brain Normal Life Content (Self-imposed behaviors)	Biological Responses	Psychological Dynamic Consequences
Sleep deprivation	Obsessive thoughts about sleep	Daytime somnolence
Caloric restriction	Obsessive thoughts about eating	Anxiety, interpersonal stress
Dietary restriction, i.e., vegetarian diet	B12, folate or protein deficiency	Lack of motivation or energy
Excessive exercise	Prolonged endorphin elevation	Lack of social motivation

The hard-driving, obsessive behavior of a corporate chief executive officer exemplifies self-imposed behavior. This individual often may be responsible for the lives of sometimes hundreds of thousands of employees and their families, for stockholders, and for delivering a safe and reliable product or service to the marketplace. Typically, the CEO brings work home and stays up late at night, which causes sleep deprivation. He or she usually travels frequently, resulting in social isolation and interpersonal stress. Frequently, this individual can find relief in psychotherapy that focuses on health maintenance issues and ways to balance corporate and personal priorities.

In a setting where there is normal brain function, normal content of life, and absence of neurotic behavior, individuals still may lack spirituality; the consequences of this lack may be the same as those caused by biological sources.

Normal Brain Inadequate or Nonexistent Spiritual Life	Psychological Responses	Dynamic Consequences
Values	Boredom	Poor job performance (frequent job changes in process of looking for truth)
Beliefs	Chronic fatigue	
Focus		
Motivation	Lack of motivation	
	Lack of acceptance	Divorce
	Overreactivity to minor issues	
	Chronic unhappiness	Domestic discord
	Incapacity to appreciate people or experiences	

The yuppie phenomenon exemplifies the results of inadequate or nonexistent spiritual awareness. Consider the professional, urban couple who has wealth, good physical health, fame, beautiful possessions, and a membership at an exclusive country club. Despite their financial success and security, this man and woman cannot find happiness because of the utter lack of spiritualism in their lives. They seek stimulation through travel and social activities to maintain a psychological "high," but nothing lasts. Only a spiritual focus will allow these individuals to find truth and purpose beyond materialism and empty social competition.

Formulating the Diagnosis

When patients present to a biological psychiatrist, they are asked to describe their main problem, or chief complaint. In the medical model the chief complaint is mapped into all possible behavioral clusters that might account for the problems. Then a sorting-out process occurs where the objective is to define brain dysfunction and cause of illness.

In psychiatry, medical model guidelines are used to define illness, but there can be unique meanings of the chief complaint.

Since defining illness in psychiatry involves self-reporting, psychiatry lends itself to malingering, where patients self-report false information for the purpose of secondary gain.

There are other ways the chief complaint can be confusing. An examination of the awareness array in the frontal lobe will explain potential problems with the chief complaint.

Interpreting a chief complaint *can* be complicated, but in everyday practice it is not so complex. Malingering is rare unless patients come from prison populations or are involved in disability determinations. It also is rare for a system in the body to be normal while the subjective assignment that the body is normal is missing (i.e., getting enough sleep but subjectively feeling that one has not slept.) The key question to bear in mind is: *Is there an independent generator of behavior that interferes with an individual's normal capacity?* (See Appendix P.)

Basically, there are two forms of chief complaints:

1. Normal complaint with awareness
2. Complaint stated by another person because the patient has no awareness

The following model details the diagnostic progression for the different classifications of chief complaints.

1. Normal complaint (i.e., a feeling that "something is wrong")
   * Illness not present
   * Insight not present (i.e., with sleep disorders the subjective assignment—that adequate sleep is being obtained—is absent)
   * Insight present (brain aberration)
   * Illness present
   * Insight not present (chief complaint usually is stated by another person, as in the case of manic schizophrenia)
   * Insight present (depression)
2. Normal subjective assignments without sensory input
   * Insight not present (hypochondriasis, somatization, panic attack)
   * Insight present (OCD)

In rare cases, a third category must be considered:

3. Malingering for secondary gain
   * Illness not present (sociopathy)
   * Illness present (malingerer may be unaware that any illness is present)

When the brain fails in its usual capacities, dysfunction that causes independent generators of behavior is identified in terms of:

1. behavioral clusters[8]
2. traditional psychosis
3. specific lobe dysfunction

See Appendix P for a case study.

After brain dysfunction is defined, then a systematic evaluation of the patient is made to formulate a psychiatric diagnosis.[9] Illnesses are defined by:

1. Clusters of symptoms
2. Family history
3. Age of onset
4. Course of illness
5. Laboratory measures
6. Response to medication
7. Ruling out of acquired causes of symptoms

The Williams 10-Step Evaluation Process (see "Williams 10-Step Evaluation Process" on pages 181–182) follows the open model, which is the way medical specialists approach organ system failure (Appendix Q).

If an individual is found to have a reasonable balance in life and has brain failure, the medical reasons for secondary brain failure first are ruled out. Brain failure secondary to medical causes appears the same as brain failure stemming from genetic causes. Scientific studies provide guidance for appropriate laboratory tests designed to eliminate more common illnesses that mimic primary psychiatric disorders.[10]

Because there are many factors (some of which are listed below) that may lead to an incorrect diagnosis, great care must be taken in examining all possible variables during the diagnostic process:

1. Highly varied chief complaint.
2. Form versus content—focus on the content of life versus the form of behavior.
3. Unusually sensitive individual generators of behavior that tend to dominate and obstruct behavioral clusters of signs and symptoms. An example is a depressed patient with

Williams 10-Step Evaluation Process

(This sample evaluation addresses *depression*.)

Step 1 Presentation of chief complaint: depression. A "chief complaint" is the patient's primary reason, described in the patient's own words, for being seen by a physician, i.e., "I'm depressed."

Step 2 Initiation of search for definable brain dysfunction, i.e., "Does the chief complaint fit into a behavioral cluster that defines brain dysfunction?" Review three methods of defining brain dysfunction: behavioral clusters, traditional psychosis, or specific lobe dysfunction.

Chief Complaint   DSM-IV Behavioral Cluster for Depression
Depression   (Five or more of the following symptoms have been present during the same two-week period and represent a change from previous functioning)

1. Depressed mood most of the day
2. Markedly diminished interest in all activities
3. Significant weight loss or gain
4. Insomnia or hypersomnia
5. Psychomotor agitation or retardation
6. Fatigue
7. Feelings of worthlessness, guilt
8. Diminished ability to concentrate
9. Recurrent thoughts of death, suicide

Step 3 Inquiry about family history, i.e., "Is brain dysfunction related to a genetic or primary determinant of behavior?"

Step 4 Inquiry about age at onset of depression, occurrence pattern, severity of symptoms, past psychiatric treatments/responses, psychiatric hospitalizations, i.e., Does the pattern fit a bipolar depressed pattern versus a unipolar depressed pattern?"

Step 5 Recording of medical history, performance of physical examination (including laboratory testing), determination of whether patient might have a medical disorder that is causing depression. In the presence of such disorders as multiple sclerosis, stroke and thyroid disease, depression would be considered "secondary depression" because it occurs secondary to a medical illness.

Step 6 Performance of phenomenologic Mental Status Examination (MSE) and determination of whether results show pattern that is consistent with depression in four behavioral categories.

1. Observed Behavior

     Appearance   Slightly disheveled
     Mood   Depressed
     Affect   Constricted
     Motor   Psychomotor slowing (both mind and body movements are slowed)

2. Queried Behavior
Upon direct questioning, no psychosis is elicited.
3. Cognitive Behavior
Cognitive testing reveals "decreased concentration" (i.e., trouble with serial sevens) but is otherwise unremarkable.

Conclusion: In this case, the phenomenology is consistent with clinical depression.

4. Special Considerations Physician inquires whether the patient is suicidal or homicidal. Patient admits to suicidal thoughts, a symptom consistent with the depression cluster.

Step 7 Testing for drug use (prescription, over-the-counter, illicit) and alcohol use. Patient denies use of alcohol and illicit drugs. Prescribed medications include antihistamines and over-the-counter medications, such as aspirin for headaches.

Step 8 Evaluation of psychosocial stressors, including divorce, financial problems, current illnesses, etc.

Step 9 Integration of interview and test data, creation of a working diagnosis and treatment plan.

Five-Step Approach to Treatment

Step 1 *Education of patient and family members about illness and its impact on the brain and lifestyle.*

Step 2 *Initiation of psychological therapies, if necessary.*

    Supportive   *Provides safety and support*
    Cognitive   *Provides affirmation*
    Behavioral   *Provides relaxation techniques*

Referral of a patient for psychological therapies first involves determination of illness consequences—specific illness behavior and resulting responses by patient—(as detailed below) and then application of the appropriate therapy.

    1. *Presentation of illness behavior*
    2. *Psychological response by patient*
Immediate Long-Term
  • *Magnified*
  • *Grief emotions*
  • *Demoralization*
  • *Anger*
  • *PTSD*
  • *Codependence*
  • *Learned negative behavior*
  • *Personality changes*
    3. *Dynamic response by patient*
Immediate Long-Term
  • *Arguments*
  • *Divorce*
  • *Fights*
  • *Loss of job, inability to progress in job*
  • *Marital discord*
  • *Social isolation*

Step 3 *Treatment for suicidal thoughts, as a special issue.*
Step 4 *Initiation of medical therapy.*
Step 5 *Formulation of plan for follow-up care.*

Step 10 Education of patient and family members.

severe insomnia whose insomnia problem may distract from the depressive cluster.

4. Prominent traditional psychosis that may look like schizophrenia, for example, yet may be caused by another pathological process. Another example is hypothyroidism causing auditory hallucinations.

5. Incomplete work-up for brain dysfunction and behavioral cluster that is secondary to medical illness.[11]

6. Bipolar form of the illness is masked, leading to incorrect diagnosis of unipolar disease.

Special Considerations

Beyond the basics of psychiatric diagnosis, there often are additional details—special considerations—to be reviewed. For example, because of decreased cerebral reserve, elderly patients often are more prone to brain failure than younger patients. Approximately 10 percent of medical disorders documented for elderly patients initially present as brain disorders.[12] For this reason, some clinicians (and I am one) believe that the mental status of the elderly should be included in the measurement of vital signs (i.e., pulse, temperature, blood pressure, and respiratory rate). Appendix R illustrates a case of misdiagnosis in an elderly patient.

Other situations worthy of special consideration are:

1. Questions of competency
   • legal impact
   • financial impact
   • childcare
   • medical requirements
2. Child molestation
3. Suicidal behavior
4. Homocidal behavior
5. Cases involving an insanity plea
6. Mitigating circumstances[13]

Childhood developmental history *may* play a part in the development of psychiatric illness or personality disorder. The biological psychiatrist does not focus on developmental history, however, because science has not established a connection between illness behavior and developmental traumas. It can be argued, however, that developmental experiences reinforce behaviors that might develop into illness or, in cases where patients have crystallized "core beliefs," lead to automatic negative thoughts.

For example, a young boy who is unable to overcome shyness may eventually develop social phobia because both parents are alcoholics and are emotionally and physically unavailable. Or, a mildly sociopathic adolescent grows up in a drug-infested ghetto where the environment reinforces sociopathic behavior. Evaluation in these and all other cases is based on the *history of illness* and present psychopathology.

Although our primary purpose in this chapter is to describe the *basics* of psychiatric diagnosis, it is worthwhile at this point to mention several clinical presentations that can make the diagnosis process very complex. Following is a list of a few of these instances:

1. *Overlapping syndromes* exist when two or more independent generators occur at the same time. For example, major depression and panic attacks can occur together.
2. *Interacting syndromes* occur when one condition (or syndrome) worsens another condition by creating physiological stress. There can be direct interaction between syndromes. In some cases, this can have a positive effect, as when obsessive compulsive disorder (OCD) interacts with attention deficit disorder (ADD) so that the ADD patient may be compelled to be more organized. More often, however, the interaction has a negative impact, as when panic disorder interacts with social phobia and intensifies the social phobia.
3. *Personality generators* of behavior may interact with illness behavior. For instance, an outgoing individual with social phobia may be motivated to become involved with Toastmasters (a public speaking group) while someone who is shy may be content to avoid social intercourse.
4. *Individual sensitivity to medications* can complicate diagnosis. Some individuals are so sensitive to low doses of medications that I refer to them as "homeopathic" patients. Others require extremely high doses of medication in order to achieve the desired effect.
5. *Unusual illnesses* may look like common illnesses. For example, OCD may present as a psychotic disorder because of obsessive images. Obsessive images may be mistaken as visual hallucinations.
6. *Medications* may have complex interactions with more than one generator of behavior. For example, a patient who is

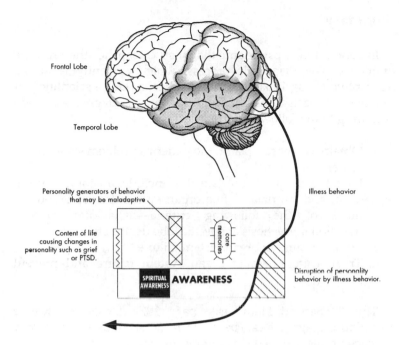

Frontal Lobe

Temporal Lobe

Personality generators of behavior
that may be maladaptive

Content of life
causing changes in
personality such as grief
or PTSD.

core memories

SPIRITUAL AWARENESS **AWARENESS**

Illness behavior

Disruption of personality
behavior by illness behavior.

Figure 8-2. Open model and the Williams Brain Model.

being treated with Prozac for depression may experience an increase in ADD because the Prozac decreases OCD.

The overall approach to evaluating special considerations involves the determination of:

1. The presence of normal brain capacities
   - Frontal lobe function
   - Executive function—directs and sustains attention, strategic thinking, decision-making, synthesis of data, working memory, change of focus of awareness (Fig. 8-2)[14]
   - Awareness function—directs subjective assignments (thoughts that are inputs to the awareness center), choice, cognizance of illness
   - Memory
   - Language
2. The absence of independent generators of behavior that would interfere with the above capacities

Summary

In conclusion, a psychiatric diagnosis establishes the presence of illness. The diagnostic process, which currently is in the descriptive phase, is based on the medical model, a scientific and rational approach to psychiatry. In general, a diagnosis is made according to the following format:

1. Obtain a chief complaint, the patient's problem stated in his or her own words.
2. Base the diagnosis on data that includes history, physical exam and lab data; define organ system failure by one or more of the following criteria—behavioral clusters, traditional psychosis or specific lobe dysfunction.
3. Look for cause of organ system failure.
4. Treat acute phase of organ system failure and prevent relapse.

The "50-Second Hour" (see page 187) details the way a psychiatric diagnosis can be made in 50 seconds in the family practice or internal medicine setting.

The open model utilizes the Williams 10-Step Approach to make a psychiatric diagnosis. The Williams Five-Part Psychiatric Plan is used to effect treatment. The overall algorithm follows:

1. Rule out psychiatric disorders, such as major depression.
2. Rule out unusual content of life, such as grief or PTSD, that can cause psychological or dynamic problems.
3. Rule out maladaptive (neurotic) behaviors.
4. Rule out spiritual issues.

Occasionally, mapping the chief complaint into a cluster of signs and symptoms may be difficult because it is not clear which cluster to map. All possible illnesses that could cause the chief complaint must be examined. For example, when the chief complaint is hallucinations, all the following illnesses could be considered:

1. Encephalopathy/delirium
2. Schizophrenia
3. Mood disorder - psychotic depression, mania with psychosis, mixed state with psychosis
4. OCD —"intrusive images"

The 50-Second Hour

The 50-Second Hour is a method of psychiatric diagnosis specifically designed for the family physician or internist who works in the traditional out-patient setting (a medical exam room simply equipped with the patient's chart). In this environment, where medical professionals typically must see as many patients as possible each day, psychotherapeutic "sessions" typically last approximately 50 minutes. (Initial appointments at the Biological Psychiatry Institute, where the environment is less rushed, last a full 60 minutes.)

Let's look at how the 50-Second Hour principle works in a specific patient exam situation.

The patient is a 50-year-old white male who presents to the internist's office with the chief complaint of low energy and lack of motivation. The patient tells the nurse that he thinks he is ill, but "I can't put my finger on the cause."

The nurse takes the patient's history, which includes complaints of progressive decrease in energy for three weeks. The patient satisfies six out of eight DSM-IV criteria for major depression. There is no personal or family history of depression. The patient drinks one to two beers per week. Review of other medical problems is negative. Although the patient relates stress at work, interpersonal and family issues are unremarkable.

The internist reviews the record of lab findings in the patient's chart, notes a history of drug abuse and performs a quick physical exam while reviewing with the patient his depressive symptoms and suicidal behavior. Based on positive behavioral clusters displayed during discussion, the internist can quickly perform a mental status exam:

The patient is a 50 year old white male who speaks in a low tone. Appearance is slightly disheveled. Manner is irritable. Mood is depressed. Affect is constricted. No overt psychosis is present. The patient is slow to respond to questions but is oriented with good memory function.

A diagnosis of major depression is made and a prescription for an antidepressant is given, with follow-up recommended 3 to 4 weeks later. The internist also encourages the patient to read *Brain Basics* so he can understand his illness, the diagnostic process, and the reason for specific types of prescribed medications.

The 50 seconds are up!

---

5. PTSD—"recurrent . . . images"
6. Temporal lobe epilepsy
7. Sleep deprivation and micro-REM (rapid eye movement)
8. Drug-induced illness, caused by prescribed medications or LSD
9. Head trauma
10. Lesions in brain, stroke, or tumor
11. Spontaneous stimulation of peripheral organ systems, i.e., when the vestibular system produces vertigo

The process of determining the differential diagnosis involves investigating all likely possibilities and finding the best fit that defines a working diagnosis. The chief complaint may not be a symptom of the behavioral illness but a *consequence* of the illness.

References

1. Psychiatry has attempted to standardize the descriptive phase through creation of the DSM-II, DSM-III, and DSM-IV.
2. Behavioral clusters previously have been described as one means of defining brain dysfunction.
3. Tomb DA. *Psychiatry*. Baltimore: Williams & Wilkins; 1995:1.
4. Tomb DA:2.
5. *Diagnostic and statistical manual of mental disorders*. 4th ed. Washington, DC: The American Psychiatric Association; 1994:32.
6. Form versus content is a constant problem in all of the major brain disorders. With major depression, the source of depression is not relevant, i.e., the physiology of the illness determines the depressive form. The same principle applies to brain disorders. For example, a woman presents with obsessive sexual thoughts that disrupt her capacity for interpersonal relationships. The patient has been treated in a sexual dysfunction clinic for five years (for the content of her obsessions). When treated for the form of her behavior (obsessive-ness), she undergoes complete remission. The major determinant is psychological, i.e., her obsessiveness, and not directed by content, i.e., sexuality.
7. In the case of sleep disorders, subjective assignment is missing, and normal reciprocal behaviors are confused. Traditionally, if individuals are tired, they can ask themselves if they're getting enough sleep. When a sleep disorder exists, although sleep is sufficient, there is no sense of being rested or of having slept adequately. The disorder actually is a subjective assignment disorder related to sleep. Patients are educated about the cause of the problem and taught how to focus on the subjective assignment of being tired, in terms of sleep adequacy.

    Hypochondriasis or somatization states occur when the subjective assignment of illness is transferred to the awareness center when, under normal circumstances, they remain only subjective assignments.

    An eating disorder is present when individuals have no subjective assignment that they are "full." In these cases, patients consume enormous amounts of food.
8. Defined in DSM-IV.
9. Hagop Akiskal notes in "Diagnosis in Psychiatry and the Mental Status Examination" that the diagnostic process in psychiatry is similar to that used in other medical specialties: personal history, family history, examination and laboratory tests comprise the essential steps. Because

the presenting information provided by patients often is so subjective, the physical exam is particularly important. A brief mental status exam also is typically included as part of the routine physical examination. (In: Winokur G, Clayton P, eds. *The medical basis of psychiatry.* Philadelphia: W B Saunders Co; 1986:370.)

10. Sternberg DE. Testing for physical illness in psychiatric patients. *Journal of Clinical Psychiatry* 1986;47:3–9.

11. Major depressive syndrome causes all syndromes to appear the same whether they are caused by a primary disorder (genetic) or secondary disorder (secondary to medical illness).

12. Alessi CA, Cassel CK. Medical evaluation and common medical problems. In: Sadovoy J, Lazarus LW, Jarvik LF, eds. *Comprehensive Review of Geriatric Psychiatry.* Washington DC: American Psychiatric Press, Inc.; 1991:171.

13. For example, individuals who have been convicted of a crime may submit psychiatric reports that describe "mitigating circumstances" that influenced the enactment of their crime, i.e., their own experience of severe sex abuse during childhood made them more prone to commit violent acts.

14. In behavioral illnesses of which patients are aware, various conditions may exist. Awareness is based on both content and form; form is based on the source of input to awareness, or a specific level in the awareness array, as illustrated below:

Awareness of a green light, while driving	Caused by outside stimulus (normal input)
Brain integrates light	Affects integration and association centers in brain (if over-stimulated, brain produces hallucinations)
Subjective assignment enters awareness center	Triggers awareness of "green" and language assignment (if overstimulated, self-stimulation or self-hypnosis results)

Also, awareness can be focused on the portion of the awareness array that governs sensitivity to color (in this case, "green"), and the awareness of green can be induced through hypnosis, for example.

If input, such as a named instinct, exceeds a certain threshold, awareness automatically focuses on that portion of the array. One example of this phenomenon is chronic pain. Patients with chronic pain may attempt to change the focus of their awareness to other parts of the awareness array to avoid enhancing the effects of pain. A second example is obsessive thoughts about eating. An underweight fashion model who observes a low-calorie diet below her hypothalamic "set point" will be obsessed by thoughts of food. The awareness center maintains this focus until instinctual needs are satisfied.

9
The Mental Status Examination

The truth is, the science of Nature has been already too long made only a work of the brain and the fancy: It is now high time that it should return to the plainness and soundness of observations on material and obvious things.

Robert Hooke
Micrographia

The medical model of psychiatry attempts to counter fads by the systematic use of scientific tools.

Robert A. Williams, M.D.

We see what we are *taught* to see. Since most of us are not taught to recognize brain failure, it is not surprising that more than 75 percent of brain dysfunction is never detected. The Mental Status Examination (MSE) is a systematic method of teaching people how to view overt behavior at a given time in order to determine the presence of brain failure. It also can help those in nonmedical professions (i.e., lawyers, counselors, ministers) take a more proactive role in applying the principles of *Brain Basics* to their professions, to more accurately assess brain function, and encourage affected individuals to seek appropriate treatment.

The MSE is the accepted method of examination and evaluation for the brain—the organ system of behavior—through the observation of overt behavior. As part of a respiratory exam, for example, an internist listens in all lung fields for abnormal lung sounds that would reveal obstruction or disease. As part of a cardiac exam, the cardiologist may tap the chest to see if there is an enlarged heart or to look for enlarged neck veins that might indicate congestive heart failure. As part of a mental status examination the neurologist or psychiatrist administers the MSE to establish the presence of brain failure.

As part of any medical evaluation, the MSE becomes meaningful only in the context of a complete physical/neurological and psychiatric evaluation. The MSE measures the mental state of the brain *at the time of the observation*.[1,2] It is an assessment of the brain in "idle" mode and does not measure how the brain functions at work, under stressful/complex conditions or in creative situations. The MSE is directed toward looking at behavior and defining either brain dysfunction or brain aberrations. By sampling different generators, the MSE provides a composite of behavior at a given time.

The usefulness of the MSE goes beyond its diagnostic implications in that it also is used in the clinical setting as a follow-up tool to monitor the presence of illness. Patients who have an illness that intersects their awareness center have the capacity to self-monitor for illness behavior. When patients return for follow-up care, the MSE is used to confirm their complaints and self-monitoring (Fig. 9-1).

The MSE assumes greater importance when illness does not intersect the awareness center. Since patients in this situation cannot see their illness, feedback to them is essential in order to promote external awareness; the MSE provides a systematic way to provide this feedback.

Despite its usefulness in many situations, the MSE is limited in several respects as well. For example, it does not take into account historical data, such as recent hallucinations, suicidal thoughts or rapid behavioral changes. If the MSE is not used within a diagnostic schema, erroneous conclusions may result.

It also is unfortunate that there is no universally accepted standard for the MSE, unlike other types of medical tests (i.e., urinalyses or electrocardiograms). Therefore, I have designed my own MSE parameters that focus on the three ways in which brain failure can be clinically defined through evaluation of the primary presentations of failure (see page 47).

The goal of a psychiatric evaluation is to provide a diagnosis and treatment plan. *The MSE alone does not yield a diagnosis.* Rather, the MSE is one step in the 10-step diagnostic process (see Chapter 8) that may help to define illness. Because the MSE can change over time, as is true for cyclical or environmentally influenced illnesses, *a normal MSE does not necessarily mean that brain failure is absent.*

Basic MSE Concepts

The psychiatric interview includes the MSE and a data-gathering mission during which historical data is systematically recorded. This information is added to a general

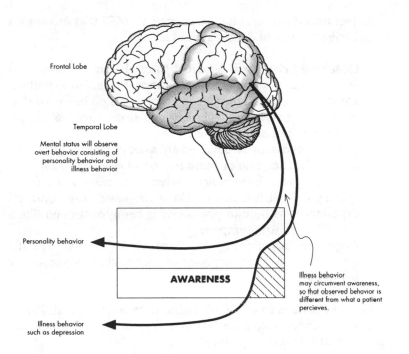

Frontal Lobe

Temporal Lobe

Mental status will observe
overt behavior consisting of
personality behavior and
illness behavior

Personality behavior

AWARENESS

Illness behavior
may circumvent awareness,
so that observed behavior is
different from what a patient
percieves.

Illness behavior
such as depression

Figure 9-1. Williams Brain Model and awareness.

database that includes results of the physical and neurological examinations.

Observations made during the MSE should separate form from content. You may recall that form relates to *physiology* of the brain, while content relates to *psychology* of the brain. For instance, if depressed mood and guilt are observed, it is important to note the form of depressed mood and guilt, not those elements about which individuals feel depressed or guilty.

Content reflects individual experience and cultural learning. To illustrate, an Australian bushman with a brain tumor might hallucinate and see an antelope, whereas a Madison Avenue ad-man with a similar tumor might hallucinate and see a fashion model. In this case, the form of behavior—a visual hallucination—is the significant element because it relates to a pathological process (an interaction between the brain tumor and the brain). The content, consisting of an antelope or a fashion model, is interesting but not meaningful.

As mentioned earlier, I have designed an MSE that focuses on three basic methods of defining brain failure:

1. **Observed behavior** is obtained through active observation and includes observation of appearance, mood/affect/anxiety level, and motor level. Emphasis is on behavior that might be related to *behavioral clusters*, such as major depression or panic disorder.

2. **Queried behavior** is obtained by asking general questions that might elicit one or more *traditional psychoses*. Examples are: "Do you hear voices when no one is around?" (perceptual disturbance) "Do you have any unusual experiences as though your body is being controlled like a robot?" (first rank symptom)

3. **Cognitive functioning** is obtained by asking specific questions on a standardized exam that might relate to *specific lobe dysfunction*.

Fig. 9-2 provides an outline of elements tested by the MSE, and Fig. 9-3 describes cognitive tests for regions of the brain and specific dysfunctions they reveal.

Observed Behavior

In observing and talking with a patient during the first phase of evaluation, remarkable features in specific areas are noted:

- Appearance: age, race, sex, body type,[3] dress, hygiene, state of health, manner
- Mood level and affect
- Motor level, marked by fast or slow movements

Past behavior reflects on current appearance, health, and hygiene, as well as on projection about how we want others to see us in the future. For instance, a depressed and suicidal patient may appear disheveled because he or she cannot visualize any future and believes appearance is irrelevant.[4] Following is an example of the exam notes a biological psychiatrist might make, based on this portion of the MSE:

Mental Status Exam

Outline of behavioral elements to be assessed

Observed Behavior
(Assessment objective - identification of specific disorder (i.e., anxiety or depression)
that may relate to a behavioral cluster)

    I.   General Appearance
        a. Age, race, sex, body type
        b. State of consciousness, manner (i.e., anxious manner)
        c. General health, hygiene, grooming

    II. Motor Behavior
        a. Gait
        b. Activity (i.e. hypoactivity or hyperactivity)

    III. Affect/Mood
        a. Stability
        b. Quality or appropriateness of mood (i.e. depressed or manic

Queried Behavior
(Assessment objective - identification of specific types of disorders)

    IV. Thought Processes (reflective of possible language disorders)
        a. Rate and pressure of speech
        b. Thought disorders (i.e., tangential)

    V. Belief Processes (reflective of possible belief, or apophany, disorders)
        a. Delusional mood
        b. Delusions

    VI. Perceptual Processes (reflective of possible perceptual psychosis)
        a. Hallucinations
        b. Illusions

    VII. First Rank Processes (reflective of possible experiential disorders)
        a. Thought broadcasting
        b. Delusional perceptions
        c. Experiences of influence
        d. Experiences of alienations

Cognitive Function
(Assessment objective - identification of cognition level)
    VIII. Mini-Mental Status Exam (30-point evaluation)

Figure 9-2. Elements of the Mental Status Exam.

A 25-year-old white male, ectomorphic, dresses neatly, healthy appearing[5] who speaks in a friendly, cooperative and appropriate manner.

Overview of Cognitive Function Tests

Following are examples of cognitive function tests that relate to different lobes of the brain. A more extensive can be found in The Neuropsychiatric Mental Status Examination by Michael Alan Taylor, M.D. (see endnote 1, Chapter VII)

Brain Region	Task	Dysfunction
Frontal Lobes	1. Global orientation	Disorientation*
	2. Draw circle	Motor perseveration
	3. Serial 7's	Poor concentration*
	4. Similarities	Poor abstract thinking
	5. Identification of upside-down objects	Disability in active perception
	6. "No if's, and's or but's;" "Methodist Episcopal"	Broca's aphasia* (dominant lobe only)
	7. Repeat word series	Immediate recall*
Dominant Parietal Lobe	1. Calculations	Acalculia
	2. Finger identification	Finger agnosia
	3. Reading	Alexia (dyslexia)*
	4. Writing	Agraphia (dysgraphia)*
Non-Dominant Parietal	1. Copy outline of simple shapes	Construction apraxia (intersecting pentagons)*
Dominant Temporal Lobe Lateral Temporo-parietal region	1. Name simple objects	Aonomia*
	2. Speech	Wernicke's aphasia
Deep	1. Recall word series	Short-term memory
	2. Relate recent events	Recent memory
	3. Recall past events	Long-term memory (all verbal memory)
Non-Dominant Temporal Lobe	1. Repeat rhythms	Poor rhythm perception
	2. Repeat and recognize musical tones	Amusia
Occipital Lobes	1. Identification of camouflaged objects	Poor visual perception

Figure 9-3. Overview of cognitive function tests.

"Mood level" simply refers to the patient's mood and whether it appears depressed, normal, or euphoric. Affect is the emotional reactivity to thoughts expressed or questions asked. Following is an example of exam notes, based on this portion of the MSE:

The patient's mood is euthymic (normal) and affect is full range. Anxiety level is low.

"Motor level" refers to the amount of physical movement that can be observed when the patient is not engaged in a motor task. Depressed patients tend to move slowly while manic patients usually are characterized by a high degree of activity, such as pacing. Following is an example of exam notes, based on this portion of the MSE:

The patient's motor level is normal.

Conversation during this phase of the MSE focuses on the patient's chief complaint, inquiries about *behavioral clusters*, psychiatric and medical history, drug and addiction history, current medication intake and family history. Behavior is observed while the physician obtains basic information from the patient.

Queried Behavior

During the second phase of the MSE more directed questions are asked about the patient's thoughts, beliefs, perceptions, and experiences. This is done in order to determine the presence of a *traditional psychosis*, of which there are four types:

1. Formal thought disorders, as reflected in higher language disorders. Receptive and expressive language is intact.
2. Perceptual disturbances, as seen with hallucinations.
3. Belief disturbances, as seen with delusions.
4. Disorders of experience, as seen when an individual feels as though his or her body is being controlled by outside forces.

Formal thought disorders, reflected through language, are evaluated during normal conversation, not any specific line of questioning. It is important to note that the *form* of language, not the *content*, is the essential element to monitor during this phase of testing—*how* an individual speaks, not necessarily *what* he or she says. For example, a manic patient will speak rapidly and change topics, whereas a depressive patient will speak in a slow, hesitant manner.

Formal thought disorders are higher order language disorders, not just language receptive or language expressive disorders. Expressive or receptive problems can be ruled out by asking a patient to repeat simple phrases, such as "The President lives in Washington" or "Methodist Episcopal." If a patient has trouble hearing (receptive) or trouble speaking (expressive), then formal thought disorders cannot be evaluated.

Neurologists perform similar sensory motor function tests to determine the presence of praxias and to rule out input or output problems. In order to measure praxias, patients are asked to perform higher order motor functions, such as demonstrating the use of a key or hammer. If patients have a sensory abnormality, such as difficulty feeling an object or motor/muscle weakness, then praxias cannot be tested.

Formal thought disorders are evaluated by asking patients direct questions. Descriptions of three of the most common formal thought disorders follow:

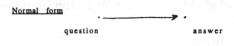

Tangential thoughts—characterized by responses where the patient talks around the main point and never arrives at the answer.

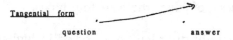

Circumstantial thoughts—characterized by responses that address the point but include excessive wording or irrelevant information. Commonly seen in elderly patients with senile dementia.

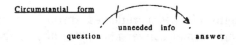

Derailment—characterized by rapidly jumping from one idea to the next. Commonly seen in manic patients, as part of flight of ideas.

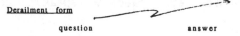

Following is an example of exam notes, based on this portion of the MSE:

Speech is normal rate without formal thought disorder.

Perceptual disturbances are marked by hallucinations in any or all of the five senses—touch, taste, smell, hearing, and sight. A hallucination is the activation of a subjective assignment of one or more of the senses when there is no corresponding sensory input. Usually, the content of a hallucination is not important. The hallucination itself, or the *form* of behavior, indicates brain dysfunction.

Nearly all illnesses can be characterized by perceptual disturbances. For example, it is logical that depression (triggered by activation of the limbic system) often is accompanied by auditory hallucinations (triggered by activation of the temporal lobe, part of which is included in the limbic system). This explains why very depressed individuals might exhibit auditory hallucinations that "convince" them they are "bad" and deserve to die.

The method of evaluative questioning for perceptual disturbances involves making inquiries about specific perceptual modalities, i.e.:

- Have you heard voices when there is no one around you? (auditory)
- Have you seen "things" that you cannot explain? (visual)
- Have you had unusual feelings in your body or extremities, as though someone is touching you? (tactile)
- Have you sensed any unusual smells that you cannot explain? (olfactory)
- Have you experienced any unusual tastes that you cannot explain? (gustatory)

Following is an example of exam notes, based on this portion of the MSE:

No perceptual disturbances noted (if answers for sensory input questions are negative).

Belief disturbances, or delusions (also referred to as "aphophanous phenomena"), occur commonly in psychiatric disorders. The neurology or neuromechanism of belief is not well described. Basically, beliefs that are not known to be false and are in line with socially acceptable beliefs are "normal."

Viewed as a system, the neurology of belief is dynamic; it has the capacity to change. Viewed on an individual basis, people have varying capacities to modify their beliefs.

Originating in the temporal lobes, belief generators of behavior are memories that involve the grouping of information or concepts into categories of "true" and "not true." Belief generators of behavior also provide memory of beliefs and have an impact on the following:

1. Perception
2. Understanding
3. Experience
4. Social learning (social matrix)

As is true of types of human behavior, belief behavior can assume different forms:

- *Maladaptive belief behavior* involves beliefs that are not known to be false but are intensely defended and often are accompanied by behavioral response that is maladaptive. An example of this would be an individual who believes in defending environmental issues so passionately that other parts of his or her life are compromised. Maladaptive belief system problems can lead to demoralization, distrust or suspicious thoughts.
- *Deviant belief behavior* takes the form of beliefs that are not false but deviate from social norms or socially acceptable beliefs.
- *Fixed false belief behavior* takes the form of delusions. In the normal realm of human behavior, there is a wide variation in the capacity to change belief systems (belief system fluidity). Individuals with delusions are incapable of changing their beliefs, however, despite the presence of real evidence to convince them to do so. Delusions indicate brain failure and are not specific for any psychiatric illness.

Following is an example of exam notes, based on this portion of the MSE:

No aphophanous phenomena elicited, or No delusions noted.

Disorders of experience, or first rank symptoms (FRS), are marked by abnormal experiences. For example, normal experiences include love and hate; individuals with FRS have experiences that are not normal, such as feeling that their bodies are being controlled like robots.

An FRS is one of the traditional psychoses and represents brain dysfunction. In the early days of psychiatry, an FRS was believed to be diagnostic of schizophrenia, but it is now known that it indicates nonspecific brain failure, not a particular diagnosis.

In evaluating disorders of experience, the following types of questions are used:

- Have you had any unusual experiences, such as the feeling that your body is being controlled like a robot (experiences of influencing)?
- Have you had any unusual experiences, such as your thoughts leaving your head like radio waves (thought broadcasting)?
- Have you had any unusual experiences that make you feel as though your thoughts are not really your own (insertion)?

Following is an example of exam notes, based on this portion of the MSE:

No first rank symptoms noted.

Cognitive functioning

The third phase of the MSE tests cognitive functioning, or the ability to perform mental tasks. It is the most objective portion of the examination because it utilizes standardized tests, such as the Mini Mental State test. This is a 30-point standardized measurement that is especially effective in testing many (but not all) cognitive functions, including memory, orientation, sequencing capacity (serial 7s), reading, writing, and ability to follow instructions. A score of 25 or more points on the mini state test is "normal."[9]

Following is an example of exam notes, based on this portion of the MSE:

Mini Mental Status Exam equals 30/30.

In summary, notes from a normal MSE would read as follows:

Psychiatric exam reveals a 25-year-old white male who is ectomorphic, dresses neatly, and is healthy appearing. The patient speaks in a friendly, cooperative, and appropriate manner. The patient's mood is euthymic and affect is full range. Anxiety level is low. The patient's motor level is normal. Speech is normal rate without formal thought disorder. No perceptual disturbance noted. No delusions noted. No first rank symptoms noted. Mini mental status exam equals 30/30.

Samples of Exam Notes

Following are examination notes, based on MSE testing, that describe five types of brain disorders:[10]

1. Alcohol withdrawal
2. Major depression
3. Hypomania
4. Dementia
5. Schizophrenia

Alcohol Withdrawal

Discussion of Symptoms
Patients with alcohol withdrawal usually experience anxiety, tremor, sweating, and irritable mood. Alcohol withdrawal stimulates the autonomic nervous system, leading to increased heart rate and sometimes sexual stimulation (which may lead to inappropriate sexual behavior).

The individual going through alcohol withdrawal appears slightly disheveled because he may have gotten up late with a hangover. As he approaches his office door, he finds it difficult to put his key in the door because of hand tremors. During the workday he complains that people are working too slowly and takes two aspirin for his throbbing headache. His secretary fears talking with him because his temper is so explosive. He shouts at her, "Get in here! Where are my sales figures?!" Later, he may make sexually suggestive remarks to her.

Conversational MSE

A 45-year-old white male presents in the medical office; he is endomorphic, disheveled, and gray-looking, speaks in a hostile manner, and is sexually inappropriate. His mood is irritable and affect is constricted. Anxiety level is high. Speech is rapid without formal thought disorder. No overt psychosis is present. He is oriented to time and place with good memory function.

Note

Withdrawal of a substance like alcohol creates a clinical effect that is opposite of the calming, sedative effect the substance produces on initial use. The clinical picture of mild alcohol withdrawal is activation of nervous system, hypertension, anxiety, tremor, sweating, increased sexuality, and irritability. In an advanced state, alcohol withdrawal can cause delirium (agitation and hallucinations) and seizures.

Major Depression

Discussion of Symptoms

Symptoms seen on the DSM-IV criteria for major depression[11] are easy to recognize in casual conversation, as the following dialogue demonstrates (O = Observer; DI = Depressed Individual):

O: "How are you doing?"
DI: "I'm down in the dumps and can't enjoy anything!" [Criteria (1) and (2)]
O: "How is your wife?"
DI: "We don't get along any more." [Criterion (c) - impairment in functioning]
O: "We ought to get together soon and do something fun."
DI: "No, I get too tired and feel guilty about not working." [Criteria (6) and (7)].

After a short conversation it is not difficult to see how five out of nine criteria could be obtained for a behavioral cluster, indicating "major depression."

Conversational MSE

A 45-year-old white male presents in the office; he is mesomorphic, slightly disheveled, hygiene is not at par with his normal level, and he speaks slowly [Criteria (1)] in an irritable manner. His mood is depressed and affect is constricted. He has psychomotor retardation (slow speech/slow movement) [Criteria (5)]. Anxiety level is moderate. His motor level is slow. No formal thought disorder is detected. No overt psychosis is noted. He is alert and oriented to time and place with good memory function.

Note

The first part of the conversational MSE brings out the patient's depressed mood and psychomotor retardation. At this point, the observer might ask about other criteria in the major depressive cluster.

Hypomania

Discussion of Symptoms

Symptoms of hypomania are easy to recognize, based on the DSM-IV criteria, as the following dialogue reveals (O = Observer; HI = Hypomanic Individual):

O: "How are you doing?"

HI: "I'm doing what every genius does [Criterion (1)], write poetry. I've been up all night writing [Criteria (6) and (2)]. I just bought a new car and plan to buy a new house [Criterion (7)]."

O: (who is having trouble getting a word in edgewise) "What are . . .?"

HI: "Let's go jogging or, no, on second thought, I'd better get a copyright [Criterion (4)]."

Note

The unusual behavior seen in hypomanics is not recognized by patients themselves because they lack insight. (A psychotherapist would call this "denial.") The behavior circumvents awareness.

Conversational MSE

A 28-year-old white male presents in the office; he is disheveled, dirty in appearance, and speaks in a rapid manner. He has pressured speech (difficult to interrupt). His mood is elevated. Affect is constricted. His motor level is increased. He has psychomotor activation. No overt psychosis is noted, but patient is unaware of inappropriateness. He is alert, oriented to time, place and person.

Note
The conversational MSE for hypomania is easy to comprehend; manic individuals are grandiose in mood and talk a great deal. They usually are characterized as being "hyper." Typically, they show very little insight into the inappropriateness of their behavior.

Dementia

Discussion of Symptoms
The first signs of dementia include forgetfulness and a tendency to get lost. The risk for dementia increases with age. A casual conversation with someone who is demented might sound something like this (O = Observer; DI = Demented Individual):

O: "What are you doing today?"
DI: "I don't remember what we have planned."
O: "How do you feel?"
DI: "I feel with my hands!" (frontal lobe sign, i.e., concreteness)
O: "Is your car in good working condition?"
DI: "My car is the one that Mr. Wilson bought; it works well, but I get lost when I drive." (circumstantial speech)
O: "Do you know the date?"
DI: "I've had many dates in my time."

Note
Conversation with a demented individual can be frustrating because of circumstantial and concrete thinking.

Conversational MSE
A 68-year-old white female presents in the office; she is neat in appearance and speaks in a slightly disinhibited and concrete manner. Her health is good but hygiene is slightly reduced as her fingernails are dirty. Her mood is euthymic. Affect is slightly constricted. Her motor level is normal. Speech is circumstantial. No overt psychosis is noted. She has reduced memory function, i.e., unaware of the date.

Note

The above MSE is for a mild form of dementia. Symptoms of dementia can involve any part of the brain as the illness progresses.

Schizophrenia

Discussion of Symptoms

Schizophrenia is marked by the presence of hallucinations, delusions, and/or disorders of experience. A casual conversation between an observer and a schizophrenic individual might sound like this (O = Observer; SI = Schizophrenic Individual):

O: "How are you doing?"
SI: "I don't know."
O: "Do you enjoy visiting with friends?"
SI: "I don't know." (frontal lobe blunting)
O: "Do you hear voices when no one is around?"
SI: "Yes, all the time."
O: "Tell me about them."
SI: "They tell me to watch out for what I'm saying to others."
O: "Do you have any other unusual experiences?"
SI: "I have thoughts that leave my head like radio waves that you can read!" (temporal lobe activation)

Note

In schizophrenia, frontal lobe blunting and temporal lobe activation are observed. When a young patient has an isolated psychosis, the source of the psychosis is schizophrenia and/or drug-induced (i.e., LSD, PCP, or psilocybin). Drugs can cause a "psychosis secondary to drug use;" schizophrenia is a "primary psychosis," due to genetic determinants.

Conversational MSE

A 19-year-old white ectomorphic male presents in the office; he speaks in a timid manner. Clothes are noncolor coordinated and he appears disheveled. Hygiene is poor. Mood is euthymic. Affect is blunted. Social skills are poor. Motor level is normal. Patient appears suspicious, looking about in a random fashion. Patient complains of hearing voices when no one is around, being suspicious that someone is going to harm him, and feeling that thoughts are leaving his head like radio waves. Speech is sparse so that normal conversation is impossible to maintain. Patient is oriented with good memory function.

Note
The MSE for the schizophrenic patient brings out an isolated psychosis (temporal lobe) with emotional blunting (frontal lobe).

Summary

In review, the Mental Status Examination is a systematic method of observing overt behavior of the brain at a given time. Its purpose is to establish the presence of brain dysfunction, not to formulate a diagnosis. During the observation stage, mood and affective abnormalities are noted that may reveal behavioral clusters indicative of brain failure. During the queried stage, the presence of traditional psychosis may become evident, indicating brain failure. When abnormalities are found during the cognitive functioning stage, specific lobe dysfunction usually is present.

References

1. Taylor MA. *The Neuropsychiatric Mental Status Examination.* New York: Spectrum Publication, Inc.; 1989:2.
2. Observation is based on activity that actually can be viewed, not on belief or subjective interpretation. For example, two physicians are observing the same patient who is sitting in a corner, talking to himself, masturbating in public, and putting in his mouth various objects he finds around him. He appears completely unaware of the activities around him.
    One of the psychiatrists is quick to *interpret* the patient's behavior, and he remarks, "This man has regressed." The second psychiatrist sees the following behaviors: abnormal sexual behavior, orality, and unusual placidity. He shows the patient a fountain pen and asks him to name it, but the patient cannot do so until he *feels* it. Only then does the physician interpret his observations to suggest that the patient is suffering from Kluver-Bucy syndrome, which indicates bilateral temporal lobe lesions.
3. Ectomorphic = thin build; Mesomorphic = average build; Endomorphic = heavy build.
4. It should be noted that appearance does not necessarily reflect an individual's *own* behavior. For instance, an Alzheimer's patient may have a caretaker who helps the patient maintain a neat, hygienic appearance. If appearance were left to the patient, however, he or she likely would be disheveled and unwashed.

5. Although the content is not important, when compared to the form, the content of a manic's speech also may be flamboyant ("I am God!") and the content of a depressive patient's speech may be self-deprecating ("I am guilty of all the world's sins.").

6. See *The Neuropsychiatric Mental Status Examination* by Taylor for descriptions of other types of thought disorders.

7. In instances of psychotic depression there is an exception to the "form vs. content" rule. Patients who have depressive content as part of their auditory hallucinations (i.e., mood-congruent psychosis) make better progress with treatment as compared to those who do not have depressive content as part of their auditory hallucinations (i.e., mood-incongruent psychosis).
Examples:

   • *Mood-congruent:* A depressed woman who has auditory hallucinations that advise her that she is a "bad" person and deserves to die, has mood-congruent hallucinations.

   • *Mood-incongruent:* A depressed woman who has auditory hallucinations that advise her that "the men from outer space have landed," has mood-incongruent hallucinations. The content of the hallucination is not depressive in nature.

8. Folstein MF, Folstein SE, McHugh PR. "Mini-Mental State": a practical method for grading the cognitive state of patients for the clinician. *Journal of Psychiatr Res* 1975; 12:196–198.

9. Although these and most other disorders have a major impact on the MSE outcome, two illnesses—panic disorder and obsessive compulsive disorder (OCD)—are difficult to detect through the MSE. Unless a patient with panic disorder experiences a panic attack during the MSE, the exam may be normal. A patient with OCD may manifest no obsessive behavior during the MSE.

10. DSM-IV: 327.

11. DSM-IV: 338.

10
Treatments for Brain Disorders

Healing is a matter of time, but it is sometimes also a matter of opportunity.

Hippocrates
Precepts

In modern psychiatry, aggressive treatment of brain disorders to prevent progression of illness is a matter of opportunity.

Robert A. Williams, M.D.

Diagnosis Based on Scientific Study

Determining the diagnosis is the most important factor in formulating a treatment plan or specific course of therapy for brain disorders. This process is based largely on identifying specific determinants of behavior, which can be biological, psychological, or spiritual in origin.[1]

In psychiatry, more than in any other medical discipline, time is a major ingredient in medical treatment. With brain disorders, the best treatment opportunity is at the beginning of the illness. In fact, medical science eventually will make many mental illnesses obsolete by treating them *before* they start.

Fig. 10-1 provides a general view of the ways in which treatments can be applied to illness behavior generated by brain disorders. In the case of illness behavior, activity is generated independent of the personality and interferes with the normal capacities within the personality structure. Treatment, which is mainly medical, is aimed at reestablishing a chemical balance within the sick neurons creating the illness behavior and stopping the production of behavior that interferes with personality behavior.

Maladaptive behavior disrupts normal human functioning (i.e., personal, interpersonal, social, or industrial activity). Within the personality structure maladaptive behavior is treated with psychotherapy, which helps individuals behave more adaptively. When unusual content-of-life affects an individual,

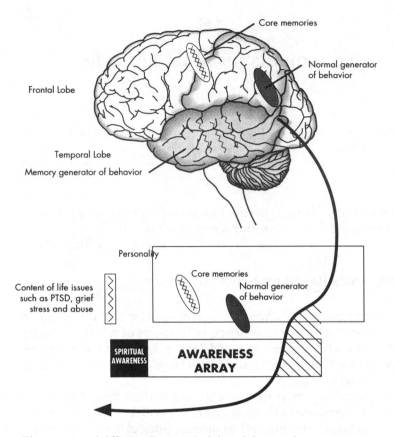

Figure 10-1. Williams Brain Model and focus of treatment.

psychotherapy is used to deal with grief, Posttraumatic Stress Disorder (PTSD), abuse, and other issues. When lack of spirituality causes behavioral problems, an individual typically is referred for spiritual awareness counseling.

As explained earlier, the consequences of illness depend on the intensity of illness and its duration. The same can be said of treatment modalities. In order to illustrate this point, let's look at the consequences of and treatment for major depression in its progressive stages of intensity:

> *Illness behavior: Major depression*
> Acute phase[2] (consequences of major depression)
> Problem: Argument with spouse or boss, secondary to
>   irritability

Consequence: Grief over loss of marriage or job, secondary to illness
Treatment: Medical intervention

Chronic phase (consequences of major depression)
Problem: Divorce or loss of job, secondary to depression
Consequence: Social isolation (because of divorce) or demoralization,
              secondary to loss of job
Treatment: Psychotherapy and medical intervention

Long-term personality changes (secondary to chronic depression)
Problem: Core memories, secondary to repeated failures
Consequence: Learned helplessness, secondary to repeated failures
Treatment: Psychotherapy and medical intervention

Many therapists say they are "eclectic" in that they utilize a combination of treatments as an approach to therapy. For mild cases of behavioral problems, "eclectic" approaches are effective, but for more severe forms of behavioral problems, it does not work well. "Eclectic" therapists tend to be biased toward a preferred mode of therapy. With more severe forms of behavioral problems, a systematic approach to defining the determinants of a behavioral problem is needed to direct more focused and aggressive therapy.

For example, the Biological Psychiatry Institute receives many referrals from psychologists who try psychological therapeutic techniques that fail. Psychologists may feel comfortable with psychological treatment styles, but psychological treatment may not be appropriate. After a largely unsuccessful course of treatment, when it is clear that the patient's behavioral determinants are biologically based, he or she may be referred to medically oriented treatment. While it is reasonable to use an eclectic approach to diagnosis, considering all major contributors to behavior, treatment should be specific and include diagnostic and treatment adjustments as required.[3]

As we have learned here, psychiatric diagnosis must be based on the medical model. Unfortunately, with alarming frequency it is based on cultural "fads" (i.e., family origin, child abuse, codependency, and others) a fact that can have tragic results in many instances. Following are several key questions to ask with regard to separating fad from scientific fact:

1. What is the scientific validation of events, such as child abuse, associated with adult illness?
2. Has illness been defined in relation to scientific study or is the behavior being studied as a symptom of everyday life? If illness is not present, therapy may bring relief to a symptom

of everyday life, but relief does not mean therapy is effective in treating illness.

3. Has the psychopathological process been defined in a way that allows it to be tested, i.e., what is the definition of codependence? Fads may help some people deal with problems of life, but treatment based on fad diagnoses have not been shown to be effective in treating medical illnesses affecting the brain.

4. Is treatment based on seeking truth, possibly challenging old theories, and making change accordingly. For example, it was a widely held "fact" for centuries that the earth was flat because it *looked* flat; scientific study has proven otherwise.

Now that the case has been made for the significance of scientific diagnosis in psychiatry, let us model the remainder of Chapter 10 on the Williams Five-Step Approach to Treatment (for the medical model):[4]

Step 1	Education of patient and family
Step 2	Initiation of psychological therapy, if necessary:
	• Supportive: provides safety, supports
	• Cognitive: provides affirmation
	• Behavioral: provides relaxation techniques
Step 3	Initiation of medical therapy
Step 4	Treatment for suicidal thoughts, as special issue
Step 5	Formulation of follow-up care plan

Step 1—Education of Patient and Family

The purpose of educating patients and their family members about brain disorders—before treatment begins and during its administration—is to promote their sense of independence and empowerment. First in the educational process is helping individuals understand brain failure and the specific ways in which it affects behavior (i.e., use of the Williams Brain Model).[5] Discussion with regard to the particular challenges of psychiatric treatment (listed below) should be a significant part of the educational process:

1. Physicians and other professionals are not trained in school or any other environment to understand behavior.

2. Very few people understand behavior well enough to help or support those with brain failure.

3. Patients with brain disorders frequently lack the capacity to see illness within themselves and, thus, do not seek treatment. Two elements, usually associated with depression and suicidal thoughts, may lead to this lack of perception.

- *Hopelessness* is the perception that the future is dim, i.e., there is no light at the end of the tunnel. The patient thinks, "If there is no hope, why see a doctor? Why take my medication? Why go on?"
- *Helplessness* is the perception that there is no ability to think or perform a task. A strong sense of helplessness renders an individual incapable of seeking help.[6]

4. Fads distract people from seeking help.
5. Psychological therapy may be incorrectly applied to biologically determined behavior, or biological therapy may be inappropriately applied to psychological problems.
6. Illness that masquerades as another illness may prevent treatment.[7]

As discussed in prior chapters, patients may not have the capacity to differentiate between illness behavior and personality behavior. Also, as previously illustrated by the Williams Brain Model, illness behavior may circumvent awareness either partially or entirely.

The second step in educating patients and family members is to help them learn to recognize illness behavior; this is not always possible. For example, many patients have had depression or residual depression for so long that they and their families believe depression is normal. Depression is *not* normal.

Patients and their families must be taught to classify behavior in two ways. One classification represents personality, or normal behavior (refer to the Williams Brain Model). The other classification represents illness, or behavior that leaves the physiological matrix of personality and creates behavior independently. As patients respond to medication, it is easier for them to recognize illness behavior; behavior that responds to medication *is* illness behavior. The number-one clue in identifying illness behavior is that it is *not* under the control of will or self-control; rather, it controls the patient and is not subject to rational thought.[8] When patients and their families can recognize symptoms that signal illness (i.e., insomnia, decreased or increased appetite, increased alcohol consumption, increased irritability), they can feel more confident about seeking medical help early in the process.

It is important for patients and their families to be taught that treatments for brain disorders do not necessarily have to be medically oriented. For example, if a patient is suffering from mild stress, he or she may elect to follow a diet/vitamin/exercise program and get more rest. Even if the main determinant is biologically based—as stress is—the treatment plan of choice could include relaxation exercises and supportive psychotherapy.

Also, it is important for patients and their families to be informed about various treatment options. If an illness worsens or does not respond to psychotherapy, medical treatment can be implemented as in the case of an individual who has been experiencing mild stress syndrome but needs medication to enhance relaxation.

Step 2—Psychological Therapies

All behavior has a mechanism of brain physiology, but it is not the scope of this book to review all psychotherapies and neuropsychiatric mechanisms.

Here's an overview of various psychological therapies, based on the neuropsychiatric model:

Counseling is an educational process to provide information to patients and address multiple issues, such as those relating to family, addiction, interpersonal, and illness. As a form of therapy used in treating *all* illness, counseling is not directed at illness itself but is designed to help patients develop treatment strategies and more informed expectations about treatment.

For example, during the counseling process a patient being treated for major depression is taught the disease symptoms. The brain stores that information, and by maintaining a heightened awareness of illness behavior, executive function can decide whether or not illness behavior is present.

Psychotherapy is a category of therapy in which the mind itself is the major determinant of behavioral change. Taking several different forms, psychotherapy involves thinking, talking, and/or interacting with a therapist or others for treatment purposes. In the biological psychiatrist's office, psychotherapy is used primarily for education and support.

As an illustration, let's look at the way in which a psychotherapist might use insight therapy to help a patient with stress syndrome.

Executive function has several ways to cope with stress, also known as "coping" or "defense" mechanisms. It can temporarily disconnect the desirable memory (resulting in repressed memory) or completely disconnect it (causing amnesia). Ignoring the memory results in denial while temporarily disconnecting feelings about the memory causes detachment.

When executive function is overwhelmed by stress, suicidal thoughts may occur as a mechanism for survival. Suicidal thoughts, although never acted upon by most individuals, have an adaptable function when life feels like it is "too much."

In summary, executive function has capacities to cope with stress through repression, amnesia, denial, detachment, and suicidal thoughts. If coping mechanisms are being used maladaptively, a psychotherapist can use insight therapy techniques to encourage changes that will result in adaptive behavioral patterns. In this case, insight is awareness that certain defense mechanisms are being used maladaptively.

Although most psychotherapists blend the use of the different types of psychotherapy—cognitive, behavioral, and interpersonal —let's examine each of them on an individual basis.

Cognitive therapy was developed by Aaron T. Beck, who theorizes that an individual's mood is determined by thoughts and ideas. In other words, modifying "thought elements" changes mood.[9]

The cognitive approach is valid from a biological perspective because it is standardized and has been tested under scientific conditions. From a theoretical point of view, the cognitive approach also makes sense. For example, an individual with mild depression experiences a plethora of negative thoughts related to prior depressions. If the negative thoughts are not countered, a cascade effect may occur, resulting in a progressive depression.

Applications of the cognitive approach are utilized in biological psychiatry. For instance, maintaining a flexible schedule of medications is an important supplement to medical therapy. When a patient detects illness behavior through the awareness center, the illness behavior (i.e., thoughts of hopelessness) can be intentionally replaced by positive thoughts, such as, "I have increased my medication and I am going to get better."

In addition, cognitive therapy can be helpful in teaching patients how to differentiate illness behavior from behavior relating to personality. Separating the self from illness behavior—depersonalizing it—lessens the negative impact of the behavior and helps patients replace negative thoughts with positive ones.

Behavioral therapy focuses on maladaptive behavior, such as isolative behavior, resistance to change and demoralization. The emphasis is on "unlearning" poor behavioral habits by setting achievable goals and working toward them gradually. For example, a common consequence of chronic depression is learned helplessness. With the help of a therapist, patients can unlearn the sense of helplessness by defining realistic goals.

Interpersonal therapy emphasizes social relationship and communication skills by focusing on the dynamic behavior between two or more individuals. This form of therapy emphasizes social relationships and communication skills. For example, consider a female patient who has bulimia and, despite medical treatments, still exercises excessively. The lengthy periods of time she spends at the gym are interpreted by her husband as rejection or that she prefers spending time exercising than being with him. The interpersonal therapist would clarify the "real" motives by facilitating communication between the bulimic woman and her husband.

In summary, psychotherapy may involve teaching problem-solving and communication techniques, stress management, setting boundaries/priorities, self-esteem enhancement, assertiveness, and interpersonal/family/social dynamics. Attitudes, values, and learned behavior patterns affect how individuals deal with life. Examining the past in terms of positive and negative experiences may yield an improved perspective with which to meet the future. Good health habits, such as adequate sleep, exercise, and nutritious diet also play an essential role in maximizing the success of psychotherapy.

Psychoanalysis, or analysis, is based on dealing with "unconscious conflicts" that impair normal brain function. Typically, the patient undergoing analysis sees an analyst, or specialist, two or more times a week, often for many years. During an analysis session the patient lies on a couch and the analyst sits off to the side, out of the patient's field of vision.

Analytic therapy is nondirective, just opposite to the highly directed medical approach to therapy. Patients in analysis are encouraged to let their executive function and memory function "float," turning off sensory distractions. Theoretically, thoughts and behaviors that arise are free from defense mechanisms, paving the way for self-discovery, expansion of the self and interpersonal growth.

There is a great difference between analysis and psychotherapy; each has its place, depending on the patient's problems. Psychotherapy is directed at making defense mechanisms more adaptable. Analysis requires more effort, a longer investment of time and is designed to allow the patient to look at the self and associated parts of the awareness array without defense mechanisms in an attempt to resolve unconscious conflicts.

When comparing psychotherapy with medical therapy, some studies on depression show that psychotherapy is as effective as medical therapy and statistically has a more sustained effect. Unfortunately, the dichotomy of psychiatry itself leads to the conclusion that psychotherapy is better or more valid than medical treatments. Studies involving more severe forms of depression, however, show medical treatments far superior to psychotherapy.

In fact, neither medical nor psychological treatments should be excluded or minimized. Rather, the choice of treatment can depend entirely on the severity of the illness and determinants of behavior in question. The primary treatment for mild depression, for example, is psychotherapy or medication, or both. The primary treatment for severe depression is medication or electroconvulsive therapy (ECT). Hospitalization as a form of treatment may be necessary to protect the patient from suicide and provide basic shelter and nutrition.

Step 3—Medical Therapies

At various times in psychiatric history, medical treatments have dominated the specialty. During the 1930s, electroconvulsive therapy (ECT) was used to treat psychosis but was nonspecific in controlling it.[10] With the advent of antipsychotic and antidepressant medications in the 1950s and 1960s, ECT became a fairly unpopular means of treatment.[11] In the 1970s, use of modified ECT (given under anesthesia and relaxation therapy) was found to be safe and effective to treat patients who did not respond to medications.

Another successful medical treatment is the use of bright light, which is used effectively to treat winter depressions (frequently associated with bipolar disorder), also known as "seasonal affective disorder." Bright light also is used to treat sleep disorders, such as delayed sleep phase disorder.

Treating a psychiatric patient with medical therapy can be a complex task. The following evaluative steps can serve to simplify the process.

1. Analyze positive effects, i.e., reduction or elimination of target symptoms of illness.
2. Determine usual side-effects, i.e., indigestion, dry mouth, tremors, sedation, insomnia, agitation, anxiety.
3. Determine idiosyncratic reactions (unusual side-effects), such as allergies that might decrease white blood count.
4. Study negative interaction with other illnesses, i.e., antidepressants may precipitate mania, may aggravate high blood pressure or addiction.[12]
5. Consider possibility that certain medications (i.e., benzodiazepines, amphetamines and narcotics) may create an addictive illness.
6. Measure possible interaction with other medications or food substances. For example, monoamine oxidase inhibitors (MAOIs), which are enzymes in the brain that break down neurotransmitters, may cause severe hypertensive crisis (high blood pressure) if used with certain foods or medications. The family of neurotransmitters known as monoamines includes serotonin, dopamine and norepinephrine. There are two types of drug interactions:[13]

   • *Pharmacodynamic interactions* occur when one drug amplifies or diminishes the effect produced by the mechanism of action of another drug.
   • Pharmacokinetic interactions occur when the effect of one drug alters the pharmacokinetics of another, leading to a change in its effective concentration at its site(s) of action.

7. Study positive interaction with other illnesses, i.e., the antihistamine effects of some antidepressants may help allergies or gastric ulcers.
8. Consider the possibility that the patient may have underlying vulnerability that has never before been manifest for a particular illness. A particular medication could bring out the underlying illness. (i.e., Lupus can be brought out by Tegretol, an anticonvulsant used for mood stabilization.)

During the neuropsychiatric follow-up appointment, an abbreviated evaluation of medications is used for practical purposes:

1. Evaluation of behavioral targets (illness behavior)
2. Evaluation of side-effects
3. Evaluation of interaction with behavioral generators of behavior

4. Evaluation of pharmacodynamic and pharmacokinetic (drug-drug) interactions

As discussed in Chapter 8, there are numerous elements that can complicate an accurate diagnosis, all of which may ultimately cause difficulty with treatment. Examples of several of these challenging diagnoses and their unique accompanying approaches to treatment are described below:

1. *Hidden bipolar disorder:* Although a patient may have no recorded history of bipolar disorder or mania, lack of response to an antidepressant can be corrected by adding lithium to the antidepressant.
2. *Overlapping syndromes:* A patient may have, for example, obsessive compulsive disorder (OCD) and bipolar disorder-mania, but treatment of OCD may aggravate the mania. Therefore, careful treatment of both syndromes is needed.
3. *Individual sensitivities to medication:* Very small doses of medication will suffice for individuals who are sensitive to medication. If larger doses are given, severe side-effects may occur. On the other hand, some individuals require very large amounts of medication, indicating an inherently low sensitivity to medication and side-effects.
4. *Hidden medical disorders:* If a patient with hypothyroidism, for example, is treated with an antidepressant, it is unlikely that the antidepressant will be effective without administration of a thyroid supplement.

The three most commonly diagnosed and treated biological disorders (see Chapter 6) are schizophrenia, mood disorders, and anxiety disorders. Schizophrenia is treated with antipsychotics, mood disorders are treated with antidepressants and mood stabilizers, and anxiety disorders are treated with benzodiazepines and antidepressants.

In the early days of antipsychotics and antidepressants, these medications were only partially effective and were comprised primarily of triyclic antidepressants (TCAs) and Thorazine-like antipsychotic compounds. The antipsychotics were nonspecific but effective in controlling most psychoses. TCAs[14] are avoided now because of their long-term effects, which cause rapid cycling of moods (more than four mood swings per year), weight gain, dry mouth, constipation, and other symptoms. The main drawback with antipsychotics then and still today is their severe side-effects, such as involuntary movements, slowed movements, and emotional and cognitive blunting (i.e., abnormal movements and difficulty in thinking).

In 1970 lithium[15] was approved in the United States for treatment of acute mania. Four years later it was approved for maintenance use to prevent mania. Lithium is specific for the treatment of manic depressive illness and has a limited number of side-effects.[16] Its use has helped promote major change in psychiatry, refuting the old concept that psychosis is specific to schizophrenia, because many patients who were believed at one time to be schizophrenic have responded positively to lithium. Even hallucinations, or catatonia, once thought to be characteristic of schizophrenia, responded to lithium. Finally, many patients once thought to be schizophrenic were rediagnosed as manic depressive.[17]

Lithium is at least equivalent to other antidepressants in treating depression in bipolar depressed patients and actually has four advantages:

1. It does not induce manic symptoms.
2. It does not induce an increase in cycling rate of moods.
3. It is well established as a preventive for depression.
4. It has established antisuicidal potential.

Because lithium is inexpensive and not well understood outside the psychiatric community, it is not heavily marketed by pharmaceutical companies.

In general, the newer antidepressants have fewer side-effects than TCAs but have no greater antidepressant effects. In the case of overdose, newer antidepressants are not lethal, while TCA overdoses can be fatal.

The action mechanism of antidepressants involves neurotransmitters and neuroreceptors previously described. For instance, Prozac, a prototype of the newer antidepressants, inhibits the reuptake of serotonin in the brain's synaptic cleft, which makes serotonin more readily available. The action mechanism of lithium involves the internal mechanisms of brain cells, i.e., secondary messengers. Primary messengers are the neurotransmitters and neuroreceptors. It is believed by most psychiatric specialists that antidepressant effects are a result of effects on primary and secondary messengers.

The permissive theory describes the effect of serotonin as a modulator of behavioral generators.[18] Note that serotonin cells are grouped in the median raphe nucleus in the brain stem. Serotonin cells project to other areas of the brain by their long axons.

A serotonin enhancer, such as Prozac, affects a variety of generators of behavior, all of which must exist in balance to maintain good health. For instance, in Parkinson's disease, it has been shown that there is a balance between the cholinergic system and the dopamine system. When disease causes a decrease in dopamine, there is a relative increase in cholinergic activity. By giving a Parkinson's patient an anticholinergic medication, a better balance will occur and the patient will experience fewer Parkinson's symptoms.

Different types of behavior also must remain in balance, as illustrated by the relationship between Attention Deficit Disorder (ADD), a dopamine generator of behavior, and Obsessive Compulsive Disorder (OCD), a serotonin generator of behavior. If Prozac or a serotonin drug enhances serotonin and decreases obsessiveness, then depending on the balance, an increase in distractedness (ADD) may occur. In other words, Prozac can upset the balance between the dopamine system and serotonin system. When Prozac is used to treat depression and yields ADD symptoms, a dopamine enhancer—such as Ritalin—may be necessary. Prozac also may aggravate tremors associated with Parkinson's disease by upsetting the dopamine/serotonin balance.

The use of Prozac as a general "life enhancer" has been proposed. This concept of a "life enhancer" can be applied to a treatment situation when *no* specific targets of behavior are present, i.e.:

1. no independent generators of behavior exist.
2. there is no unusual content in an individual's life
3. there are no strong generators of behavior (related to personality) that are maladaptive.

The proposal notes that Prozac would not be used to treat illness but would enhance basic personality. The use of Prozac for this purpose is irrational, as the balance of all generators of behavior represent the total personality. Changing the balance of generators of behavior serves no purpose and may create behavioral abnormalities.

Generally, mood disorders are divided into two categories of treatment: (a) bipolar mood disorders are treated with mood stabilizers, such as lithium, valproic acid, and Tegretol.[19] Frequently, however, mood stabilizers do not provide adequate antidepressant effects for bipolar depressed states, so antidepressants are needed to augment these medications, and (b) unipolar mood disorders are treated with antidepressants, such as Prozac and Wellbutrin.

Approaches to psychiatric treatment varies widely, of course, according to individual attitude and style of practice, based on training and experience. Informed patients can choose a style of medical care that fits their personal need and philosophy. The use of benzodiazepines in the treatment of anxiety disorder is a good example of how treatment styles differ.

Benzodiazepines belong to a family of medications that affects specific receptors in the brain (benzodiazepine receptors). Valium was the first diazepine discovered and others marketed since then include Xanax, Ativan, and Librium. Klonopin[20] is a long-acting benzodiazepine with low side-effects that is commonly used to treat anxiety attacks.

The side-effects of benzodiazepines are many, but the two that cause the most concern are sedation (which can impair driving or the use of heavy equipment) and addiction (which is a concern for all medications with addiction potential).

Patients who have a history of being chemically dependent have vulnerable addiction generators of behavior and should not be given benzodiazepines, or great caution should be taken in prescribing them. However, according to Robert DuPont, "Patients who are *not* chemically dependent and are given a benzodiazepine as part of medical treatment do *not* become addicted. Furthermore, DuPont states, " [The] distinction we must make is between physical dependence and addiction. There *is* no relationship between physical dependence and addiction."

Some physicians rule out the use of all medications that have addiction potential, while others rule out the use of only benzodiazepines because of possible benzodiazepine addiction (sometimes called "benzophobia" or fear of the use of benzodiazepines). First-hand experience with the horrors of benzodiazepine addiction greatly influences physician attitude toward benzodiazepine use.

The addiction model for benzodiazepines is the same as for any addiction. Benzodiazepines interact with vulnerable addiction generators of behavior and create a desire for benzodiazepines that exists independent of personality behavior. Withdrawal of benzodiazepines yields a temporary physiological response to decreasing or discontinuing benzodiazepine use.

There are four phases in the medical treatment of a psychiatric disorder.

1. *Survival:* protection of a patient who may be suicidal or accident-prone.
2. *Treatment of target symptoms:* direct treatment, for example, of anxiety or insomnia.
3. *Treatment of underlying illness:* use of a medication, such as lithium, to stabilize underlying mood.
4. *Prevention of relapse:* use of medications to maintain stability of health.

It is not within the scope of a general text like *Brain Basics* to elaborate on all aspects of psychiatric treatment; this is far too complex an area of study and one that is constantly changing. Following is a descriptive overview for each of the four phases of medical treatment.

Medical treatment based on aspects of survival[21]

Symptom	Treatment
1. Suicidal thoughts derived From illness behavior	1. Hospitalization—to provide protection 2. Electroconvulsive therapy (ECT)—to provide quick relief from suicidal thoughts 3. Benzodiazepines—to reduce anxiety/agitation associated with suicidal thoughts 4. Education, support, and cognitive therapy—to assist patients to cope with suicidal thoughts
2. Poor judgment that might lead to accidents	1. Hospitalization—to provide protection 2. Temporary restriction from driving 3. Home convalescence with supervision—to avoid accidents 4. Supervised care in convalescence facility
3. Inability to care for basic needs, such as food, shelter and personal hygiene (often seen in catatonic states or during bouts of severe illness)	1. ECT—to provide rapid normalization 2. Hospitalization—to provide global support until patient is well enough for self-care

Medical treatments based on target symptoms

Symptom	Treatment
1. Insomnia—as a result of other illness and/or antidepressant side-effects may cause a sleep deprivation syndrome. Sleep deprivation is a stressor on brain function and adds "fuel to the fire" of illness	1. Soporifics, such as Desenyl (mild sedating antidepressant)[22] or Ambien (sleeping medication)[23]
2. Anxiety/agitation—a form of psychic pain. Just as time must pass in order for an antibiotic to relieve the pain of pneumonia, so time must pass in order for an antidepressant (or other psychotropic) to relieve the pain of anxiety	1. Ativan[24]

Medical treatments based on underlying illness (those commonly treated at the Biological Psychiatry Institute, detailed in Chapter 6)

Disorder	Treatment
1. Mood disorder	1. ECT for severe or treatment-resistant mood disorders (see "How Electroconvulsive Therapy Works," on page 225) 2. Lithium/Depakote/Tegretol for bipolar mood disorder 3. Antidepressants, such as Prozac, Paxil, Wellbutrin or Effexor, for unipolar depression
2. Panic disorder	1. Benzodiazepines, such as Klonopin, or antidepressants, such as Tofranil, Prozac, Zoloft or Paxil
3. Obsessive compulsive disorder (OCD)	1. Serotonin reuptake blockers, such as Anafranil, Prozac, Luvox, Zoloft and Paxil
4. Schizophrenia	1. Antipsychotics, such as Zyprexa or Risperdal
5. Dementia	1. Search/test for correctable causes of illness, provide treatment for specific symptoms as follows: Depression—same as for mood disorder described above Psychosis—same as for schizo-phrenia described above Memory loss—cholinergic enhancer,[25] such as Aricept[26]

How Electroconvulsive Therapy (ECT) Works

Electroconvulsive therapy (ECT) is the safest and most effective treatment in psychiatry for catatonia, psychotic depression, severe mania, suicidal thoughts, treatment-resistant depression, severe mood disorders in pregnant women, and others. This form of treatment is used to eliminate symptoms while medication or maintenance ECT is used to prevent relapse. Unfortunately, ECT is underutilized because of the stigma typically associated with it and, possibly, its cost. Side effects may include mild headache that lasts for a few hours and temporary memory impairment. Treatments are administered two or three times per week and generally yield an average improvement rate of 10 to 20 percent per treatment. Thus, 5 to 10 treatments usually are required.

The ECT treatment team consists of the treating physician, the anesthesiologist or nurse anesthetist, and the treatment nurse. While the patient is relaxed and under anesthesia, a low-voltage electrical current is applied to one or both temples, which causes a local affect of decreasing the seizure threshold. (Stimulation of one side of the head is called unilateral electrode placement; stimulation of both sides is called bilateral electrode placement.) Seizures are *induced* with the electrical current and occur spontaneously because of internal brain mechanisms. All brains have the capacity to experience seizures, most running their course in 20 to 60 seconds. After the anesthesia is metabolized within a few minutes, the patient awakens.

Side effects of unilateral treatment are less pronounced than bilateral in that there is less temporary memory impairment. Bilateral treatment, however, is more effective in the treatment of mania, and 70 to 80 percent of the time is more effective in the treatment of depression.

Medical treatments based on underlying illness (those not commonly treated at the Biological Psychiatry Institute, detailed in Chapter 7)

Disorder	Treatment
1. Addiction	There is no medical treatment for addiction; treatment follows 12-step program described in Chapter 7. Treatment team may include a sponsor, psychologists, a biological psychiatrist and addiction specialists. Comorbid conditions that predispose to addiction relapse and withdrawal symptoms are treated medically.
	Most addiction treatment programs take a comprehensive view of all possible determin-

ants of substance use (see
Chapter 5). The following
diagram illustrates a comprehensive view of determinants
for alcohol use.

Determinants for Alcohol Use (with the potential for addiction)

Social Determinants	Psychological Determinants	Self-Medication of Biological Disorder	Addiction Determinants
Elements that promote alcohol consumption: 12-step program can be supplemented with halfway house therapy, group therapy, other social support systems designed to maintain sobriety.	Childhood abuse, PTSD, grief over losses, resentments, women's issues. Group or individual therapy (under direction of psychologist) provides strategies to cope with stress	Treatment for this narrow focus should be provided by a biological psychiatrist	See "Social Determinants"

2. Attention deficit disorder (ADD)
  Psychostimulants, such as Dexedrine, Ritalin, and Cylert.

3. Sleep disorders
  Chronobiology (resetting of the clock by progressive sleep times), use of melatonin at nightand light therapy during daylight hours

4. Eating disorders
  Bulimia nervosa is treatable with desipramine or Prozac; there is no satisfactory medical treatment for anorexia nervosa

5. Social phobia
  Best treated with monoamine oxidase inhibitors (MAOIs), such as Nardil or Parnate. Other helpful medications are Prozac and Klonopin.

Appendix S provides a listing of commonly prescribed psychiatric medications. Appendix T provides an example of how a treatment team works together in treating the various symptoms present in a menopausal, bipolar patient with a history of diabetes.

Follow-up care designed to prevent relapse

Five variables can contribute to medical relapse of illness:

1. cycling of illness

2. seasonal effects
3. hormones
4. stress
5. other illnesses

If a patient detects active illness through self-monitoring, each of the above variables is evaluated.

Treatment response time in psychiatry is slow, with most antidepressants having maximum effect in 3 to 6 weeks. (For example, lithium may take 4 to 8 weeks, or longer, to yield results.) Occasionally, patients respond in 24 hours, but this is the exception, not the rule.[27]

When an individual is ill, waiting any length of time for improvement is an agonizing process. For this reason it is essential that psychiatrists provide psychological support, either directly and/or through referrals to therapists.

Step 4—Treatment for Suicidal Thoughts

Up to 10 percent of patients who are suicidal also are homicidal, so that in these cases brain failure can cause death for the patient and significant harm for others. Clinically, the biological psychiatrist must weigh the positives and negatives with the patient in order to decide which medications to use.

Step 5—Follow-Up Care

Tracking patient progress is vital to the psychiatric treatment process, so regular follow-up visits with the physician who is directing treatment are very important. The psychiatric specialist may use the following "checklist" to review patient status during follow-up visits (Fig. 10-2).

1. Confirmation/review of current medications—patients frequently change or forget to take their medications or make mistakes in dosages.
2. Review of effects of medication—a review of the Williams Brain Model and medication targets is important for self-monitoring. The use of mood charts to plot the result of self-monitoring can be helpful. Mood charts help assess effectiveness of medications and predict seasonal affects/cycling patterns of illness.

Patient's Name:_____
Diagnosis: _____
Referral: _____
Date: _____
The patient is a _____ year old _____ who
returns for a medication followup. The current medications are:

The following clinical effects are reported:

Current life stressors are:

PSYCHIATRIC EXAM: Reveals a _____ year old _____
who speaks in a _____manner. Appearance is _____.
Mood is _____. Affect is _____. Motor level
is _____. Psychosis including first rank symptoms,
perceptual disturbances, and aphophanous phenomena are _____.
Cognitive fuunctioning including memory and orientation is

_____.

Laboratory Values

Neurological Exam:Weight: /
                                        Blood Pressure: sitting:
                                                          standing:
                                        Pulse

Reveals a _____ appearing _____.
Gait is normobased with good associated arm movements.
Outstretched arms reveal _____ . Finger to nose
is _____. Extraocular movements are full
without nystagmus. Pupils are _____ and react to light.
Motor tone is _____. Reflexes including biceps,
brachiodialis, petellar and achilles are _____ and
_____. Anxiety level is _____.
Suicide risk is _____.

Assessment :

Plan   Diagnostic:
          Theraputic:

Figure 10-2. Outpatient medication follow-up.

3. Analysis of psychosocial stressors—a review of stressors is important as a determinant of behavior.
4. Psychiatric examination—see Mental Status Exam (Chapter 9).
5. Neurologic assessment.
6. Assessment of control of illness.
7. Plan:
   • diagnostic considerations
   • therapeutic considerations
   • educational considerations, including self-monitoring

The most important step in follow-up care is education of the patient. This process includes:

1. Review of the Williams Brain Model
2. Discussion with regard to target symptoms and time frame for recovery.
3. Discussion with regard to self-monitoring guidelines.
4. Description of ways to respond to illness symptoms in the event of relapse.
5. Review of health maintenance issues, such as diet, exercise, sleep, resources for coping with stress and avoidance of drugs/alcohol for self-medication purposes.

Summary

The treatment of psychiatric disorders is based on a systematic diagnosis based on determinants of behavior. Treatment of illness is based on the Williams Five-Step Approach:

Step 1   Education of patient and family
Step 2   Initiation of psychological therapy, if necessary
Step 3   Initiation of medical therapy
Step 4   Treatment of suicidal thoughts, as special issue
Step 5   Formulation of follow-up care plan

The most important focus of any treatment is, of course, survival (prevention of mortality). The remaining considerations for medical therapy (an expansion of no. 3 in the Williams Brain Model outlined above) are:

1. Treatment of target symptoms
2. Treatment of underlying illness

3. Prevention of relapse (prevention of morbidity)

Evaluation of medications involves four steps:[28]

1. Evaluation of behavioral targets (illness)
2. Evaluation of side-effects
3. Evaluation of interaction with behavioral generators of behavior
4. Evaluation of pharmacodynamic and pharmacokinetic (i.e., drug-drug) interactions

Every follow-up appointment includes the use of the following behavioral tools:

1. Review of the Williams Brain Model
2. Discussion with regard to self-monitoring guidelines
3. Discussion with regard to variables that influence mood
4. Review of possible effects of medication

Major causes of treatment resistance are:

1. Inadequate trial of medication, i.e., using too little medication or for too brief a duration
2. Presence of medical disorders that either cause new symptoms or prevent effectiveness of medication
3. Presence of overlapping syndromes, i.e., panic disorder and major depression (If all disorders are not treated, the untreated disorder will prevent the treated disorder(s) from responding

The bottom line for treatment strategies is to give patients the resources for controlling illness behavior instead of being victimized by illness behavior.

References

1. One day in the not-too-distant future, this book will be obsolete, as it is based on psychiatric treatments that target modification of specific metabolic *systems*. Soon treatments will focus on modification of enzymes and RNA/DNA composition.

2. Treatment attempts made at this stage of illness are focused on preventing illness from progressing to the chronic phase and, eventually, personality changes.

3. The writers of "General System Theory" note that, "Identification of the type and location of the pathology can indicate to the clinician the proper sorts of therapy to use. If the basic fault is in matter-energy processing, perhaps that can be corrected by diet, by drugs that effect metabolism, or by surgery that alters matter-energy flows. If the basic fault is in information processing, the clinician can use psychotherapy that alters neurotic habits that block pathological signals." (In: Freedman A, Kaplan H, Sadock B, eds. *Comprehensive Textbook of Psychiatry, II.* Baltimore: Williams & Wilkins, 1976:43.)

4. The Williams Five-Step Approach relates to the *treatment* approach to psychiatric illness.

5. The Williams Brain Model is a schematic of the brain, demonstrating illness behavior.

6. When an individual feels hopeless and/or helpless, thoughts of his/her illness dominate normal personality capacities.

7. For example, major depression in the elderly can be mistaken for senile dementia (senility) because the conditions can exist together and can produce the same symptoms. Sometimes only careful evaluation or a trial of antidepressants can separate the two. If depression is treated, the patient will improve to the level of the dementia.

8. Medical science still has no concrete answer with regard to treating "irrational behavior" or activity that is independent of personality and not within the will or self-control of an individual.

9. In his early research, Beck noted important changes in perception and reasoning associated with depression. First, Beck examined his patients' emotional reactions to personal events, and then he tried alternative ways to interpret perceptions. He placed special emphasis on acquiring skills for coping with relapse and highlighted the following progression of symptoms by which to identify illness:

    - Initial signs of illness
    - Emotional overreactivity
    - Decreased capacity to cope with stress
    - Decreased functioning

    Both emotional overreactivity and decreased capacity to cope with stress directly relate to negative thought processes.

10. ECT is a medical procedure used in treating catatonia, treatment-resistant depression, psychotic depression, and other disorders. After an extensive work-up, ECT is performed under anesthesia since it causes mild cardiovascular distress. During the ECT procedure, electrical stimuli are applied to the patient's temples, which cause the brain to begin a synchronous discharge sequence that lasts approximately 30 to 60 seconds.

Common side-effects include mild headache and temporary, short-term memory impairment. The American Psychiatric Association Task Force has found ECT to be safe, effective, and underutilized. Unfortunately, the negative stigma it bears prevents appropriate use.

11. By that point ECT had gained an unsavory reputation for abuse, as described in Ken Kesey's 1962 novel, *One Flew Over the Cuckoo's Nest*.

12. Medications can be double-edged swords. For instance, while lithium can prevent depression and suicide, if taken in overdose it can be toxic or even fatal.

13. Preskorn SH. *Clinical pharmacology of selective serotonin reuptake inhibitors*. Oklahoma: Professional Communications, Inc.; 1996:145.

14. The TCA most frequently utilized, desipramine, has a comparatively low side-effect profile.

15. Lithium is a metallic ion similar to Sodium Chloride, or table salt. It is prescribed as lithium carbonate (a soluble salt or slow-release preparation) and as lithium citrate (a liquid). Lithium is found in the body only in trace amounts but lithium treatment is not intended to treat a deficiency in the body's lithium level.

No one is sure how lithium works. Scientific studies have shown it to be effective in both eliminating symptoms and preventing relapse. Lithium alone may not be effective enough to control mood swings, but medications, such as valproic acid, Tegretol, and Nardil, may be used along with lithium to control mania.

16. Possible short-term side-effects are tremors and nausea; long-term use can cause hypothyroidism.

17. Patients with schizophrenia, anxiety disorder, and obsessive compulsive disorder do not respond to lithium.

18. Gerner RH, Bunney WE. Biological hypotheses of affective disorders. In: Berger PA, Brodie HKH, eds. *American Handbook of Psychiatry*. New York: Basic Books, Inc.; 1986:272.

19. Mood stabilizers are medications that have both antidepressant and antimanic effects. All antidepressants have the potential to aggravate or induce mania.

20. Klonopin, brand name; clonazepam, generic name.

21. There are many ways patients can die because of brain failure. Survival is the number one priority in treatment.

22. Desenyl is the brand name; trazodone is the generic name.

23. Ambien is the brand name; zolpidem is the generic name.

24. Ativan is the brand name; lorazepam is the generic name.

25. Remember, the nucleus of Mayhert (the basalis nucleus) degrades in Alzheimer's disease.

26. Aricept is the brand name; donepezil is the generic name.

27. At the Biological Psychiatry Institute, 60 percent of patients respond to medication in 1 to 3 months; 30 percent respond in 3 to 6 months; 10 percent take longer than 6 months to become stabilized.

28. This abbreviated list is used clinically. The longer list provided on page 218 of the text is used when a more comprehensive evaluation is warranted.

11
Choosing a Biological
Psychiatrist/Summary Concepts

The major task of the 20th century will be to explore the unconscious, to investigate the subsoil of the mind.

Henri Bergson
Le Rêve

The major task of the 21st century will be to explore the biological and genetic mechanisms of the brain. Good-bye to the 20th century.

Robert A. Williams, M.D.

As described in Chapter 1, toward the end of the 19th century Sir William Osler, Jr., M.D., presented the principles on which our current medical model is based. The medical model, as we have learned, emphasizes a scientific and unbiased approach to diagnosis and treatment of illness. Biological psychiatry applies Osler's principles in an attempt to avoid fads and misconceptions.

When Sigmund Freud and other psychoanalysts set forth their psychologically based models for psychiatry, American psychiatry was seduced, along with the rest of the world, by these new concepts. Tragically, the American public has been paying the price of this seduction for nearly 100 years.

My primary motivation in writing *Brain Basics* is twofold. First, I have set out to clarify the biological foundation of psychiatric disorders and help readers recognize and understand the diagnosis and treatment of brain failure. *Brain Basics* also is designed to help patients understand the nature of behavior and provide an informational interface not only between patients and physicians interested in treating brain disorders through biological means, but also between physicians and individuals in other professions. Part of this process involves informing readers how to identify and select a biological psychiatrist.

Secondly, *Brain Basics* seeks to change generally held misconceptions about mental illness. This is a challenge since only 10 percent of the public believes brain disorders are biological or brain-related.[1] Social attitudes and beliefs have created a stigma related to psychiatry and mental illness; it is my hope that *Brain Basics* can help individuals understand the scientific facts underlying psychiatry and play a significant role in redefining mental illness. *It is a fact that there is no perfect brain and that all of us will face one or more forms of brain failure at some point in our lives.*

Choosing a Biological Psychiatrist

In selecting a biological psychiatrist, begin with characteristics that traditionally are sought in a physician, regardless of medical specialty:

1. High ethical standards
2. Comfortable patient bedside manner
3. Good communication skills
4. Medical competence
5. Genuine compassion for patients
6. Enjoyment of work

Generally speaking, psychiatrists are medical doctors who participate in 4 years of post-M.D. training in behavioral science. They are authorized to prescribe medications, order laboratory tests, and conduct physical examinations. Biological psychiatrists specialize in the diagnosis and treatment of medical disorders that affect the brain. They adhere to the following principles:

1. The medical model of practice is a rational and scientific approach to understanding brain disorders.
2. There is a basic understanding of the nature of behavior, based on the following concepts:

   • Form vs. content
   • Determinants of behavior
   • Independent generators of behavior
   • Definition of brain dysfunction/psychosis/brain failure
   • Definition of illness
   • Mental status examination findings
   • Brain model dynamics

3. There is a systematic approach to the diagnosis and treatment of brain disorders.
4. Physical examination of patients is conducted during each office visit.

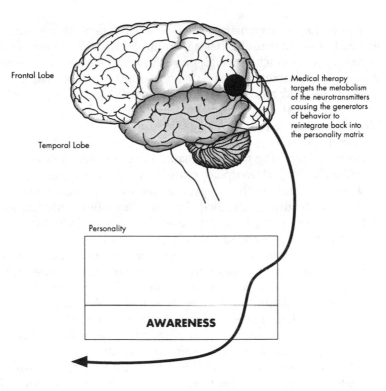

Frontal Lobe

Medical therapy targets the metabolism of the neurotransmitters causing the generators of behavior to reintegrate back into the personality matrix

Temporal Lobe

Personality

AWARENESS

Figure 11-1. Williams Brain Model.

Biological psychiatrists practice clinical medicine much as internists do. Those who seek medical care are known as "patients," not "clients." Patients are seen during "appointments," not "sessions."

Competent biological psychiatrists offer patient education programs that include:

1. Tutorials during appointments. (Each appointment should focus on principles of biological psychiatry, utilizing a simple model of the brain—as illustrated in Fig. 11-1—and emphasizing self-monitoring and prevention of relapse.)
2. Printed materials explaining illness.
3. References explaining illness.
4. Information about educational and support groups.

The biological psychiatrist's office arrangement also is much like that of an internist in that it is equipped with all the elements necessary to conduct thorough physical examinations. There is an examination table, blood pressure cuff, reflex hammer, stethoscope, opthalmoscope, and other neurological instruments. Most biological psychiatry offices are equipped with a blood-drawing station as well.

Patient examinations, including neurological assessments, are performed according to the Williams 10-Step Evaluation Process (see Chapter 8). Follow-up appointments are done systematically and may be similar to the process followed at the Biological Psychiatry Institute, detailed in the Outpatient Medication Follow-Up (see page 228). Patient evaluations are scientific and medications are prescribed only when appropriate.

In order to remain up-to-date with current progress in their specialty, biological psychiatrists refer often to scientific literature on human behavior. Models of behavior that are scientifically based serve as diagnostic and treatment examples, and research findings that define illness are used as references. Double-blind placebo-controlled studies that attempt to eliminate bias in evaluating treatment modalities also are valuable.

Those who are trying to decide if they need assistance from a biological psychiatrist should begin by asking themselves one key question—"Is the major determinant of a behavioral problem biologically based?" The following questions can be used to help formulate the answer:

1. Is a traditional psychosis present?
2. Is a behavioral cluster indicating brain failure present?
3. Are specific cognitive (thinking) deficits, such as disorientation or memory problems, noted?
4. Are there medical problems, such as stroke, diabetes, Parkinson's disease that might cause behavioral problems?
5. Does the patient take prescribed or over-the-counter medications that can cause behavioral problems?
6. Is there a family history of mental illness?
7. Does the patient abuse drugs, such as alcohol, cocaine, and others?
8. Is there a history of birth injury, prolonged bouts of fever, seizures?

If brain failure is definable, then the search for a biological psychiatrist can begin. The following questions can serve as a guideline for patients in determining the treatment philosophy of specific physicians:

1. Does the biological psychiatrist try to define brain failure?
2. Does the biological psychiatrist assess biological/psycho-social/spiritual balances?
3. Does the biological psychiatrist look at the impact of brain failure on personal/social/interpersonal/industrial functioning?
4. Does the biological psychiatrist have a systematic method of evaluation, including biological tests, neurological assessments, and assessment of family history?
5. Does the biological psychiatrist try to educate patients and family members, utilizing the Williams Brain Model? Is the emphasis on prevention and self-monitoring?
6. Is there a support system available and referral resources to help patients during the recovery process?
7. Does the biological psychiatrist have an examination room with the usual equipment, including blood pressure cuff, stethoscope, etc.?
8. Is there a biologically-trained nurse (RN) or staff who can perform tests, educate patients about medications and side-effects and offer supportive care?
9. Are there hand-outs available, informing patients about medication side-effects and illness?
10. Does the biological psychiatrist have protocols for maintenance medications and for eliminating ongoing medications?

One of the purposes of this text is to educate individuals who are confronted with behavioral problems. I have written this book as though I were talking to my patients. Most people who are faced with a behavioral problem do not get help because they do not recognize illness. Many people are faced with a nonstandardized, obsolete psychiatric care system. *Brain Basics* provides a knowledge base that will allow a healthcare consumer to make intelligent choices about psychiatric care. If a problem warrants a biological evaluation, finding a biological psychiatrist may be difficult because there are so few who are trained as such.

Summary Concepts

The basic building block of behavior, the neuron, is classified according to the primary neurotransmitter it releases. Because alteration of the neurotransmitter's metabolism causes behavioral change, therapy for illness behavior focuses on modifying or realigning this metabolic change.

Following are the major concepts presented by *Brain Basics*.

1. The **brain** is the organ system of behavior.
2. **Behavior** is anything that reflects brain activity.
3. **Overt behavior**, which is observable or experienced without special equipment, can be classified according to **form** (created by physiology of the brain) and **content** (determined by the content of one's life.)
4. **Psychosis** is any overt behavior that clearly represents brain dysfunction. Traditionally, psychosis is defined as one of four types of disorders:
   • perceptual dysfunction
   • belief disturbance
   • thought disorder
   • disorder of experience
5. **Brain dysfunction** and **psychosis** are synonymous with **brain failure**; all three terms have the same meaning.

Mental illness, or a neuropsychiatric brain disorder, is due to an inherent vulnerable generator of behavior that can interfere with normal brain function. The generator of behavior may be vulnerable because of a primary process or genetics or a secondary process, such as head trauma. Brain failure may occur as a result of external stress, such as drug use, or a metabolic process that causes delirium.

When brain failure is caused by severe stress, it is not mental illness because the primary process is not due to an inherently vulnerable generator of behavior. An important way to test whether brain failure is caused by stress is to remove the stress and determine if brain failure symptoms disappear. Brain failure, secondary to stress, is not a brain disorder but is caused by a decreased threshold for illness.

6. **Generators of behavior** are groups or systems of brain cells (neurons) that have a common function, such as memory, language, or mood.

7. **Personality** is the overlapping physiological matrix of all generators of behavior in the brain.

8. **Failure** of a generator of behavior causes predictable signs and symptoms of illness, regardless of the cause of failure.

9. **Brain failure** occurs when one or more generators of behavior produce behavior that is independent of the personality matrix and interfere with an individual's normal behavioral capacities. Brain failure is defined by three **clinical presentations**:
   - behavioral clusters
   - traditional psychosis
   - specific lobe dysfunction

10. **Illness** is caused by either genetic determinants and/or environmental/medical determinants. It is characterized by age of onset, course, behavioral clusters, mental status examination results, family history, laboratory test results, and response to medication.

11. **Biological determinants** create the form for all behavior. When evaluating a behavior problem, biological determinants of behavior are ruled out before considering other elements, such as unusual content of an individual's life, maladaptive generators of behavior related to personality, poor strategies of life and spiritual matters. Fig. 11-2 illustrates the algorithm that is used to systematically evaluate the presence of a behavioral problem.

12. **Psychiatric diagnosis** is in the descriptive phase. DSM-IV provides descriptive behavioral clusters. Formation of a psychiatric diagnosis first requires definition of brain dysfunction, then researching the source of illness. Primary brain disorders, which are genetic, are diagnosed by (a) ruling out environmental trauma or medical conditions that can mimic a primary psychiatric disorder, and (b) searching for family history that might support a primary psychiatric diagnosis. (The Williams 10-Step Method is based on this diagnostic process.)

13. **Awareness** is a sustained reflective thought. The awareness center, residing in the frontal lobes of the brain, receives subjective assignments from instinct, memory, self, sensory input, and executive function. Executive function has the capacity to direct focus within the awareness center. Awareness has a distinct place in psychiatry in that it is used to help patients monitor for the presence of illness. For patients who have no capacity for awareness, special

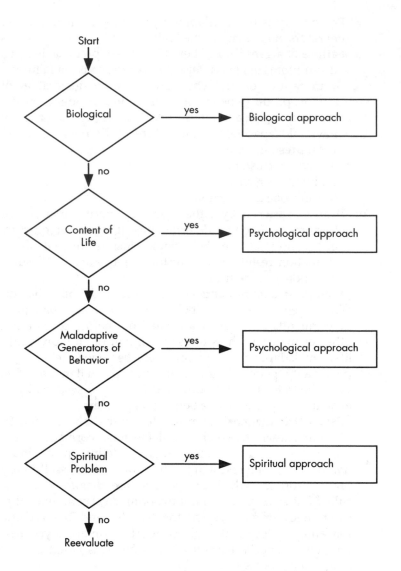

Figure 11-2. Algorithm for evaluating a behavioral problem.

considerations are applied, such as directing awareness to
the consequences of illness.
  14. **Self-monitoring** uses awareness to detect:
    • Symptoms of illness
    • Decreased capacity to cope with stress

- Emotional overreactivity
- Decreased functioning

15. **Basic determinants of behavior** are classified as biological, psychosocial, and spiritual. Biological determinants yield behavioral form; psychosocial and spiritual determinants yield behavioral content. Behavioral problems that relate to a change in form of life have a biological source. Behavioral problems that relate to a change in content of life have a psychosocial or spiritual source.

16. The **basic biological influences** on behavior, beyond genetically determined brain structure and biochemistry, are:
    - cyclical variables of illness
    - circadian stressors
    - hormones, vitamins and essential nutrients
    - psychological stressors
    - illness

17. The **consequences of mental illness** involve all possible psychological conditions, dynamic problems, and changes in personality. Early identification and treatment of brain dysfunction minimizes consequences of mental illness. Chronic illness potentially can change personality structure, which can profoundly affect treatment outcome.

The consequences of mental illness can be treated with psychotherapy and at times with both medical treatment and psychotherapy. Typically, patients are referred for psychotherapy for the following reasons:

- Grief
- Codependency
- Communication problems
- Assertiveness skills
- Strategies for dealing with life
- Posttraumatic stress disorder
- Spiritual problems
- Coping skills
- Demoralization issues
- Psychological therapies that apply to medical illness, such as OCD or addiction, or adjunctively enhance medical treatment

Following are several examples of the ways in which illness behavior can affect personality behavior, often manifested in not taking prescribed medication.

Illness	Mechanism Preventing Patient From Taking Medication
1. Mania	Patients have no capacity to "see" illness and think, "Why take medication for behavior I cannot see?"
2. Depression	Patients suffer from severe hopelessness and think, "Why take medication when the situation is hopeless?"
3. Schizophrenia	Patients suffer from severe suspiciousness and believe someone may be seeking to harm them with prescribed medication.
4. Panic disorder	Patients with severe anxiety may be unable to swallow.
5. Attention deficit disorder (ADD)	Patients have no capacity to plan ahead or to execute plans and, therefore, cannot remember to take medication.
6. Obsessive compulsive disorder (OCD)	Patients with severe obsessiveness often have trouble ever getting around to taking medication.

Fig. 11-3 provides further clarification on the ways illness behavior can affect personality by comparing patients with students in a classroom.

18. **Undesirable events** can lead to several mechanisms that can interfere with normal instinctive, sensory, and social functioning, as well as the sense of self. For example, divorce can cause the following types of problems in these areas.

Instinctive function (relationship)	Difficulty with bonding Difficulty with territoriality (setting boundaries)
Sensory function	Posttraumatic stress disorder Grief reaction
Social function	Guilt Social isolation Problems with interpersonal dynamics
Sense of self	Shame Defiance of values

There is a pattern to sitting in an audience that relates to illness.

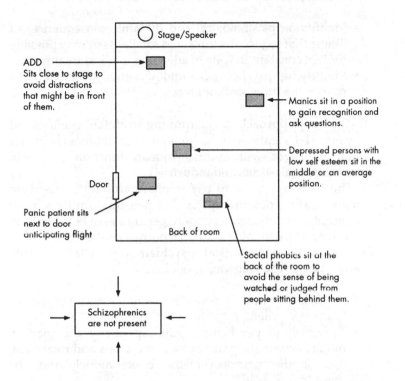

Figure 11-3. How illness affects where a person sits in a lecture room.

19. The basic **mental status examination** provides at a given time a phenomenologic exam of overt behavior. The three parts of the mental status exam target the dysfunctional brain's primary clinical presentations.

Mental Status Examination	*Target Dysfunction*
Observed behavior	Behavioral clusters
• Appearance	
• Mood/affect	
• Motor level	
Queried behavior	Traditional psychosis
Specific lobe dysfunction	Specific deficits, such as memory loss

20. **Biological psychiatric treatment** is designed to restore normal physiology of the brain so that outward behavior

reflects personality. The focus of psychotherapy, as it relates to biological treatment, involves:

- Identifying psychological and dynamic consequences of illness that reduce the threshold for illness or may possibly remain constant in spite of adequate medical treatment.
- Identifying psychological and dynamic problems that reduce the threshold for illness.

21. The basic **approach to determining treatment** is illustrated by Fig. 11-1 Treatment targets elimination of illness behavior that interferes with normal human function (i.e., self, interpersonal, social, and industrial).
22. The basic approach to **psychopharmacology** is based on manipulating neuroreceptors and neurotransmitters in an attempt to regulate independent generators of behavior and reintegrate them into the brain's normal physiology.
23. **Choice of a biological psychiatrist** should be made according to the following guidelines:

- Physician attitude ("bedside manner") and vocabulary (patient vs. client; appointment vs. session)
- Approach to psychiatry, including use of the medical model, systematic philosophy of diagnosis and treatment, use of the neuropsychiatric brain model, and the neurological exam.
- Office configuration similar to that of an internist.

In conclusion, *Brain Basics* is written for a wide variety of readers—from physicians, physician assistants, nurse practitioners, therapists, attorneys, and administrators to anyone else interested in learning about basic brain mechanisms. It provides basic psychiatric definitions, an introduction to the brain model and neuropsychiatry as well as details on brain failure, identification of brain failure, descriptions of illness and a basic model of illness. It is my hope that the knowledge gained from *Brain Basics* will help readers approach behavioral problems in a systematic and intelligent manner, using existing mental health resources in their communities.

It is my intent that *Brain Basics* be used for two main purposes: (a) to alleviate the pain resulting from mental illness, and (b) to control the generators of behavior that create illness so that individuals can enjoy life according to their God-given capacities and pursue a spiritual existence.

The process of healing involves a spirit of shared existence between physician and patient. In fact, the physician-patient relationship represents a unique spiritual bond that is focused on helping individuals with illness. Over time, as trust develops, the physician can provide hope when hope is lost, energy when energy is depleted, help when the patient is helpless. The physician's goal is to provide the spiritual awareness that can promote healing.

Robert A. Williams, M.D.

Note

If you or your organization wish to review *Brain Basics* in a seminar setting, please contact us by mail, phone, or fax:

Biological Psychiatry Institute
5133 N. Central, Suite 107
Phoenix, Arizona 85012
Phone: 602.279.1026
Fax: 602.279.0838

References

1. Following is an overview of public perceptions about the origins of mental illness, noted in Stephen Stahl's *Essential Psychopharmacology* (Cambridge, UK: Cambridge University Press, 1996:100):

71 percent	Due to emotional weakness
65 percent	Caused by bad parenting
45 percent	Victim's fault; can "will" it away
43 percent	Incurable
35 percent	Consequence of sinful behavior
10 percent	Has a biological basis; involves the brain

2. By studying the model of the brain, patients can learn how to monitor the following types of illness behavior that intersect the awareness center:

   - Symptoms of illness
   - Emotional overreactivity and decreased capacity to cope with stress
   - Decreased capacity to function

For illness that does not intersect with the awareness center, patients can monitor:

- Consequences of illness
- Feedback from other people

3. There are a few medical problems, such as addiction, that are not treated medically. Addiction to foreign substances is treated nonmedically with the 12-step program. Other conditions that have been labeled by our society as addictions (i.e., "sex addiction," "food addiction") are not truly addictions. Certainly, maladaptive sex or maladaptive use of food can be a behavioral problem, and I refer such problems for psychotherapy or for 12-step treatment. In fact, 12-step programs provide such good guidelines for behavior and life strategies that everyone would benefit from a 12-step program, regardless of illness type.

4. The challenge in dealing with patients who do not "see" their illness cannot be underestimated. At the Biological Psychiatry Institute the following guidelines are applied in an attempt to communicate with these patients:

- Educate patients about the neuropsychiatric model of the brain.
- Provide social sources of information, such as books, hand-outs, videos, and referral to educational groups. (Social matrices associated with these elements are powerful influences on belief systems in that they provide external validation of ideas.)
- Counsel patients on consequences of behavior (things they *can* see). Relate concept of "tough love."
- Utilize groups, such as family (interventionary), to influence patients' beliefs.
- Provide psychotherapy to heighten awareness of current experiences that relate to illness.
- Consider hospitalization in case patients are dangerous to themselves or others.

Retrospective

One's consciousness, which is oneself, is filled with one's own concepts and conclusions and with other people's ideas; it is filled with one's fears, anxieties and pleasures and with occasional flashes of joy and with one's sorrow. That is one's consciousness. That is the pattern of one's existence.

Krishnamurti
The Wholeness of Life

Brain Basics is an attempt to make sense out of our current knowledge of behavior. Most concepts in *Brain Basics* have been around, in one form or another, for a long time. For instance, in 1599 Ben Jonson wrote:

> Some one peculiar quality
> Doth so possess a man, that it doth draw
> All his affects, his spirits, and his powers
> In their confluctions, all to run one way.
> *Every Man in His Humour*[1]

Without intending to, this century's-old passage describes the modern-day Williams Brain Model. "All his affects, his spirits, and his powers" relates to independent generators of behavior. "Confluctions" relates to interference with normal brain capacities. "All to run one way" relates to disturbance of normal human functioning.

By extracting old ideas (such as Jonson's) and combining them with new concepts to form an understandable model, *Brain Basics* attempts to demystify and counter the societal stigma of mental illness.

All individuals will experience brain failure at some point in their lives because no brain is perfect. In many cases the instances of failure will be caused by unusual content of life issues involving grief, depression, or posttraumatic stress syndrome. It is to be expected that the powerful generators of behavior that comprise personality will, at some point, function maladaptively.

249

Simply defined, the brain is a physical organ system that generates behavior; there is nothing mystical or spiritual about it. Yet, a high degree of spirituality is required to deal with unusual content of life issues. We must learn to approach these common issues in a way that combines an intellectual understanding of the scientific medical model with spiritual awareness that exists as a product of inner serenity.

The medical model, as we have read earlier, was introduced in the 1800s by Sir William Osler, Jr., M.D. This model paved the way for the scientific diagnosis and treatment of medical disorders and is still the foundation of modern medical practice. Psychiatry, however, took a different path in the early 1900s, promoting a distinction between diagnosis and treatment of mental disorders and physical disorders.

The division of mental health and physical health into two unrelated entities has had many negative consequences for both patients and physicians. The primary result has been perpetuation of the widely held notion that patients with mental disorders are "crazy" and that they bear some sort of personal responsibility for their illness.

As explained previously, various forces contribute to the continuation of the stigma associated with mental illness. Despite the power wielded by tenured physicians in academic medicine, the legal system, insurance companies, and others—who have vested interests in maintaining psychiatry's old status quo —psychiatry is changing. This change signifies an evolution in understanding from one based on the mechanism and genetics of illness to one based on an understanding of the origins of illness. Ongoing research and education about illness origins will lead to new attitudes toward mental illness and more effective treatment.

Part of understanding the origin of illness is related to comprehending the origins of *life*. The future of psychiatry beyond genetics and behavior will involve the nature of existence. Existence is based on the physical properties of time, space, matter, and energy. The brain reflects the apparent physical domains with subjective assignments that have developed through evolution. Existence, as it is experienced by human beings, is truly a miracle.

It is difficult to imagine how our vast and complex universe (including the substance that makes up the human brain) began as a mass of elemental particles approximately the size of a volleyball. The "big bang" (theory of creation) is believed to have been followed by the creation of domains whereby the interaction of fundamental particles of matter, energy, time, and space created the ongoing nature of existence, as we perceive it.

To illustrate how perceptions of existence may change in the future, let's look at matter. According to human perception of our physical domain, matter is discrete and firm, like a genie in a bottle. In reality, matter is not fixed because it if is subjected to high energy and forced through a narrow opening, it can be converted to a wave form. The genie that appears as a discrete object is released from the bottle and takes on a wave form. Or, if matter is abruptly split apart, it may release energy.

Matter has an apparent permanency because the inherent loss of time particles is slow, compared to the clocks that impact human awareness, which move relatively quickly.

Future assumptions about the beginnings of the universe may include the following concepts:

1. According to Stephen Hawking in his book, *Stephen Hawking's Universe*, the universe began as a group of singular particles. Following the big bang of creation, the singular particles broke apart to form an array of particles. These particles interact in a way that creates reality as we know it, i.e., time, space, mass, energy, gravity, and electromagnetic radiation.

2. The release of time particles from protons is very slow, which gives mass an apparent stability. This stability allows relatively fast clocks to exist, as individuals perceive "reality."

3. Time is inherent in all things that exist. Depending on the energy state (relative speed and gravity), time particles are released at different rates (i.e., clocks can be slowed down or speeded up). For example, black holes change "mass," so that three-dimensionality does not exist.

4. Time is both relative and absolute. If time particles are crowded into one place and not allowed to be released, there is no time or reality, as we see it, i.e., a black hole or an absolute beginning. After creation, time becomes relative and inherent and, thus, independent from the beginning.

5. The human brain is a product of time (evolution), an organ system of awareness, the interplay of an array of particles that were produced by creation.

The curious and mystical aspects of brain function that relate to existence are part of the unknown frontier of psychiatric knowledge, understanding, and belief. In fact, psychiatry's task in the coming centuries will be to more accurately define existence. Today, existence in the physical sense is mass/energy/time/space. In the brain sense existence is awareness of physical being.

I have several hopes for *Brain Basics*—first, that it will be, as Dr. Jack Games stated during his review of this book, "an owner's manual for anyone with a brain"; second, that it will, in some way, help people achieve spiritualism and to celebrate the distinctive beauty of their lives; third, that readers (and eventually all mankind) may personally embrace the goodness and importance of life and follow a path based on the following unitarian principles:

- The inherent worth and dignity of every person
- Justice, equity and compassion in human relations
- Acceptance of one another and encouragement to spiritual growth in our congregations
- A free and responsible search for truth and meaning
- The right of conscience and the use of the democratic process within our congregations and in society at large
- The goal of world community with peace, liberty and justice for all
- Respect for the interdependent web of all **existence** of which we are a part

Thanks for taking the time to read *Brain Basics*. I hope it has given you practical tools with which to respond to brain dysfunction, as well as a new appreciation for the human brain as a miracle of universal evolution.

Reference

1. As quoted in C. Hugh Holman's *A Handbook to Literature* (Odyssey Press; 1960:109–110).

Appendix A
Case Study of the Impact of Attention Deficit Disorder on Employment

A 48-year-old white male has satisfied the DSM-IV criteria for Attention Deficit Disorder (ADD) since age 5. The patient has a brother with ADD who is successfully treated with Ritalin.

The patient joined a newly formed corporation at age 43. At the beginning of his career his ADD was adaptable. His creative ideas and scattered thoughts prompted other employees to think beyond traditional boundaries. As the company grew and formed sustained markets, however, the need to stay focused was essential. The patient was unable to plan and execute tasks in order to satisfy corporate demands; his ADD no longer was adaptable.

After the patient's treatment with Ritalin, he again was able to adapt to corporate needs.

Appendix B
Case Study of the Impact of Alcoholism on Employment

The patient is a 50-year-old white male who has been in sales for 25 years. Until 5 years ago, the patient was a top salesman; at that time he was affable, gregarious, and known to enjoy "wining and dining" clients. Initial use of alcohol facilitated the patient's work and his relationship with sales clients. During the past 5 years, however, overuse of alcohol has impeded his work. The patient is no longer a top salesman and is having increasing problems with other salesmen.

With a family history of alcoholism (his father), the patient satisfies the DSM-IV criteria for alcoholism and alcohol withdrawal syndrome. Through Alcoholics Anonymous the patient has attained sobriety and has gone on to be the vice president of sales in his company.

Appendix C
Case Study of the Impact of Manic Depression on Employment

The patient is a 45-year-old female who started a company at age 40. Her company sets up Web page sites. At first, the patient's seemingly boundless energy and lack of need for sleep contributed to the company's success.

As the patient's bipolar illness progressed over time, however, she cycled into depressions. Her depression caused increased need for sleep, irritability, low energy, low motivation, and low self-esteem. All the preceding traits were highly disruptive to the operation of her company.

After the patient was treated for manic depressive illness, she resumed leadership of her company.

Appendix D
Case Study of Major Depression Syndrome

A 34-year-old female presents in the month of October with depression for 1 month. The patient is employed, married with two children. The patient has no illicit drug use. Her medical history is negative except for an occasional bladder infection. The patient satisfies the DSM-IV criteria for major depression, displaying seven out of nine criteria ("depressed mood, hypersomnolence, decreased interest in most activities, fatigue, feelings of worthlessness, decreased ability to concentrate, and weight gain).

After the birth of her two children, the patient experienced mild depression. The patient has had no prior psychiatric evaluation or treatment. The patient has noticed depression during the past two winters. During high school, the patient noticed being moody after menarche. The patient also notes being very irritable and at times depressed during her premenstrual period. Her current depression affects her ability to function at home and has caused severe interpersonal stress with her husband of 10 years. In fact, divorce has been discussed on a number of occasions.

The patient functions well at work. The patient denies suicidal thoughts and has no history of suicide attempts. The patient's mother has a history of cyclic depression with one suicide attempt. Her maternal grandmother was institutionalized and given electroconvulsive therapy for depression. The patient gives a history of mild elevation of mood. The patient satisfies the DSM-IV criteria for hypomania (inflated self-esteem, decreased need for sleep, more talkativeness, shopping cycles).

On examination the patient's neurological and physical condition are normal. Psychiatric exam reveals a cooperative white female. Her manner is irritable. Her mood is moderately depressed. Affect is slightly constricted; motor level is slightly slowed. No psychosis is present, including perceptual disturbances. Cognitive functioning is normal. Mini mental status exam is 29/30.

Subsequent medical tests, including CBC, blood chemistries, UA, serum electrolyte levels, thyroid profile, and EEG, are normal.

The patient's diagnosis is bipolar disorder, depression based on early onset, history of hypomania, three causative generators of depression, postpartum depressions, and seasonal pattern. A positive response to lithium correlates with the diagnosis of bipolar disorder.

Treatment

The patient is begun on lithium carbonate with excellent antidepressant response in 3 weeks and is continued indefinitely to prevent further depression. The patient's PMS also is reduced. The patient is referred for marital counseling to help reestablish her marital relationship that was disrupted by her depressive illness.

Appendix E
Case Study of Self-Monitoring for Illness Behavior

A 40-year-old white female has history of bipolar disorder. The patient has been stable on 1200 mg of lithium carbonate for 5 years. She is married with two children and has a history of mild postpartum depressions. Occasionally, she also has premenstrual irritability. Recent stressors include purchasing a new home. The patient works as an insurance agent, and her husband is an electrical engineer. She has a good interpersonal relationship with her husband and a healthy life. Her medical problems include allergies.

The patient presents for treatment as a self-referral in the month of October with depression. She is taught how to self-monitor; internal awareness shows depressed mood, irritability, decreased capacity to enjoy people and experiences, trouble going to sleep, increased need for sleep, increased appetite with weight gain, and mild suicidal thoughts.

Discussion

The patient's self-monitoring leads to awareness of the following problems:

1. Internal awareness of symptoms that relate to illness behavior, i.e., depressive cluster
2. Difficulty in coping with problems at work
3. Excessive emotional reactivity with children (two sons)
4. Reduced quality of work

In this patient's case, a review of the checklist of elements that can influence mood reveals the presence of the following:

1. **Possible cycling of mood.** Lithium is used to prevent mood swings. The patient's lithium level is 0.7 mg (low

therapeutic); lithium carbonate is increased to 1500 mg per day.

2. **Seasonal effects.** The short autumn days may destabilize mood, so the patient is placed on light therapy (10,000 lux for 1/2 hour each morning).

3. **Hormonal imbalance.** Hormones may destabilize mood in the premenstrual period. Recent gynecological exam is normal.

4. **Stress.** The patient's recent purchase of a home is a major stressor. The following stress-reducers are suggested to the patient:

    a.   Increase exercise
    b.   Limit work, at least temporarily
    c.   Observe good dietary habits
    d.   Consult therapist for supportive therapy

5. **Allergies.** The patient is found to have active symptoms of allergy and is referred to her family physician for treatment.

Treatment

The patient is treated, using the following algorithm:

1. **Survival.** The patient is aware that her suicidal thoughts are not her thoughts and feels she can control them; she has no plan to commit suicide. She is instructed to contact, on an emergency basis, the Biological Psychiatry Institute (BPI) if she has out-of-control suicidal thoughts.

2. **Symptoms of illness.** The patient is given sleeping medicine to take temporarily, as needed, to enhance sleep.

3. **Treatment of underlying illness.** Use of lithium carbonate is increased and light is utilized to eliminate the destabilizing effects of short days. Patient is referred to family physician for allergy treatment.

4. **Prevention.** Patient is instructed in maintenance use of lithium carbonate and self-monitoring.

Follow-up self-monitoring reveals the following improvements:

1. Patient's depression ended 2 weeks after initiating treatment.

2. Internal awareness shows no symptoms of illness.
3. Patient's emotional overreactivity to her sons is gone.
4. Patient is fully functional at work.

Appendix F
Case Study of Major Depression
Secondary to Multiple Sclerosis

A 35-year-old female presents with depression. She satisfies the DSM-IV criteria for major depression. She has no family history for depression and no history of drug abuse. The patient moved from Boston to Phoenix at age 30. She has a history of two depressions during the past 3 years, both of which were accompanied by weakness, stumbling gait, and one incident of double vision.

Psychiatric exam reveals a depressed white female. Affect is slightly constricted. Motor level is slow, manner is irritable. No psychosis is present. She is alert. Mini mental status exam is 30/30.

Neurologic exam shows weakness in both arms. She has cerebellar tremor in right hand. She experiences double vision. MRI of brain shows lesions compatible with multiple sclerosis.

Treatment

The patient is diagnosed with major depression secondary to multiple sclerosis. She is treated for depression with antidepressants and referred to a neurologist specializing in MS.

Appendix G
Case Study of Major Depression
Secondary to Dementia

A 50-year-old white male presents with a 3-week history of depression. The patient is very anxious and agitated. There is no personal or family history of depression, no history of drug abuse. The patient is married, employed as an insurance agent, and has two children. He has no particular psychosocial stressors except that he always is under pressure to make insurance sales.

The patient's medical history includes a history of hypertension. Current medications include Procardia 30 XL for hypertension.

Patient satisfies the DSM-IV criteria for major depression.

Psychiatric exam reveals a mildly depressed white male. Affect is slightly constricted. No psychosis is present. Manner is nervous. The mini mental status exam is 22/30, indicating borderline dementia. No history of drug abuse. Assessment is major depression with mild dementia.

Treatment

Antidepressants are prescribed for depression, with the knowledge that, as the dementia progresses, depression will become less responsive to medications.

Appendix H
Case Study of Bipolar Depression

A 17-year-old white female high school student who had been having suicidal thoughts for two weeks is seen in the office. She awoke one morning irritable and depressed. Her mother committed suicide at age 40. She lives with her father and stepmother. She satisfies the DSM-IV criteria for major depression. She has no history of drug abuse. She maintains good grades in school and was planning to attend college. She has no psychiatric history but was depressed for 2 to 3 weeks, 1 year ago, after breaking up with her boyfriend. She has no history of PMS.

The patient has hobbies, including water-skiing. She has friends at school and belongs to the theater club there. She has good bonding with her father but has disputes with her stepmother, especially about control problems. She was brought up in a Baptist Church and goes to a Bible study on Sundays.

Physical exam and neurological exam are normal. Thyroid studies, EEG, vitamin B12 and folate, complete blood count, and blood chemistries are normal.

Treatment

The patient is treated with lithium; an antidepressant will be added if the lithium does not exert sufficient antidepressant effects. After 6 months of treatment, maintenance lithium therapy will be considered on an individual basis.

Appendix I
Case Study of Unipolar Depression

A 65-year-old married, retired male, who reports anxiety and depression for 3 months, is seen in the office. The patient has no history of depression nor does he have a family history of depression. The patient lives in a retirement community and had been active in many activities, including golf. The patient was raised as a Mormon and has maintained his faith. There is no history of alcohol or drug use. The patient satisfies the DSM-IV criteria for major depression.

Work-up, including physical exam, EEG, complete blood count, blood chemistries, vitamin B12 and folate levels, is normal. (In the elderly we look for particular evidence of strokes and tumors. Medications for high blood pressure and other illnesses also may contribute to depression.)

Treatment

The patient is started on a tricyclic antidepressant. Once the patient responds to medication, maintenance antidepressants will be considered on an individual basis after 1 year.

Appendix J
Case Study of Masked OCD

A 72-year-old white retired male presents with treatment-resistant depression. The patient, who has tried all antidepressants without success, retired at age 65 and soon thereafter began to experience depression. The patient satisfies the DSM-IV criteria for major depression. With regard to this patient's unsuccessful treatment for depression, the following factors are examined:

1. Adequate trial of antidepressants—it is concluded that the patient had many adequate trials.
2. Medical conditions that might prevent medications from working—the patient went to Mayo Clinic and received a complete neurological and medical work-up, both of which were normal.
3. Overlapping psychiatric syndromes—the patient is found to have severe obsessions, especially relative to risk aversion and severe resistance to change.

Treatment

The patient satisfies the DSM-IV criteria for obsessive-compulsive disorder. After treatment focuses on cognitive therapy for OCD, in combination with medical therapy, the patient's depression improves.

Appendix K
Case Study of Juvenile OCD

An 8-year-old white male is brought to the office with the chief complaint of "inattention." Both the mother and school teacher believe the child has attention deficit disorder (ADD). The mother reports that her child ignores her, despite repeated attempts to gain his attention. The teacher reports similar inattention, especially when the child is reading a book.

The child's performance in school is excellent, overall. In fact, the child tends to be overdevoted to homework at the expense of other activities. He also has a history of handwashing rituals. The family history for ADD is negative. The child's maternal uncle was treated for OCD. The child's mother is a perfectionist and worries a great deal. The child does not satisfy the diagnostic criteria for ADD but does satisfy the diagnostic criteria for OCD. Physical examination and laboratory tests are negative.

Psychiatric exam reveals a calm 8-year-old white male. Manner is appropriate and cooperative. Motor level is normal. Mood is euthymic. Affect is full range. No psychosis is present. The patient pays attention to all that is said (no inattention). The patient is alert-oriented with good memory function. The normal psychiatric exam is consistent with OCD.

Discussion

The educational process includes an overview of conditions that cause inattention. Because ADD is common and well known, ADD is a reflex diagnosis for many. All psychiatric diagnoses have the capacity to cause inattention. The following examples demonstrate how different diagnosis may interfere with attention.

In the case of obsessive compulsive disorder, a patient may be distracted by intrusive unwanted thoughts. In the case of schizophrenia, a patient may not be able to concentrate because of auditory hallucinations. In the case of panic disorder, a patient may have trouble planning and executing tasks because of high anticipatory anxiety.

Appendix L
Differential Diagnosis for Undefinable Psychosis

A 70-year-old white female presents with sudden onset of the complaint that "they are fooling around with my air conditioner." The patient feels that listening devices are being placed in her home air conditioner. She states, "I can hear them up there!" On numerous occasions the patient has called 911, but police inspections of her home have revealed no intruders. The patient's relatives are quite concerned and state that the abnormal behavior began about 1 month prior to her presentation at the Biological Psychiatry Institute. The patient is fixed in her belief and is in total terror about "these people," causing her insomnia because of fear. The patient states, "I know it sounds ridiculous, but it's true."

The patient has a history of heart failure and is on Lasix and Digoxin. Her blood work, including Digoxin levels and potassium, is normal. The patient's physical exam and neurological exam are normal.

The patient undergoes an MRI of the brain that shows mild ischemic changes consistent with age. The MRI shows no major stroke, aneurysm, tumor, or AV malformation.

The patient has no drug abuse history nor history of taking over-the-counter drugs. There is no history of psychiatric disorders, personality disorder, or treatment.

Psychiatric exam reveals a calm white female. Her manner s friendly and appropriate. Her dress is neat. Her health is good. Her mood is euthymic (normal). Affect is full range (normal). Her motor level is normal. Psychosis is present, as described in a previous paragraph. She is alert and oriented to time, place, and person. She scores 30 out of 30 on the mini mental status test. She does not satisfy the DSM-IV criteria for major depression or schizophrenia.

Differential Diagnosis

This elderly patient presents with an isolated delusion, sudden onset, in the setting of a normal physical and neurological exam. The differential diagnoses, or possible causes of the patient's delusions, are many:

1. Late-onset schizophrenia—patient has no history of any personality traits that would correlate with schizophrenia, such as schizoid personality
2. Drug-induced psychosis—patient has normal Digoxin levels and blood chemistries
3. Use of over-the-counter drugs—this may be a high probability, but the patient's family confirms no over-the-counter drug use
4. Substance abuse—this may be a high probability, but the patient's family confirms no alcohol or substance abuse
5. Structural lesion in the brain—MRI shows no major lesion in the brain
6. Remote effects of cancer—physical exam is normal; appetite and weight are normal
7. Thyroid disease—vitamin B12 and folate levels are normal

Discussion

Seemingly, the patient has a psychosis for no definable reason. In my opinion, the sudden onset and the MRI results showing ischemic changes (i.e., very small strokes) point to the cause. Randomly, small strokes can occur with minimal or no consequences. If, by chance, a small stroke hits a strategic part of the brain, then psychosis can result. (Strokes can cause *any* psychiatric syndrome.) With advancing age the probability of stroke increases. The patient is advised to follow the stroke prevention program (i.e., ASA, diet to control cholesterol, exercise). Later, symptoms gradually decrease without use of antipsychotics, indicating recovery from stroke.

Appendix M
Differential Diagnosis for Suspected OCD and ADD

A 16-year-old female is brought to the Biological Psychiatry Institute by her mother because of obsessive behavior. The patient has a 3 to 4 year history of obsessing about her health. Her prior physician diagnosed her as having obsessive compulsive disorder (OCD) and attention deficit disorder (ADD). The patient has a history of mood swings. The only family history is her father, who is bipolar. The patient's mood has been stabilized for 5 years with Tregretol. The patient is taking Ritalin for ADD, without effectiveness. She has no history of substance abuse.

The patient's medical and neurological exams are normal.

Psychiatric exam reveals a very nervous-appearing 16-year-old female. The patient sits holding her chest, as if in pain. Her manner is highly distractible, but friendly and cooperative. She is jumpy and squirms in her chair. Her mood is anxious. Her affect is constricted. Motor level is increased. No psychosis is present. She is alert, oriented to time, place, and person. Her mini mental status test is normal (30 out of 30).

The patient's psychiatric history includes satisfying the DSM-IV criteria for major depression and hypomania. The patient has had a good response to Tegretol in controlling her moods. It has been believed that the patient's inattentiveness, distractibility, and motor restlessness are related to ADD and that the patient's obsessive thoughts about her health are related to OCD.

Discussion

All psychiatric disorders have the capacity to cause obsessive thoughts and inattentiveness. In order to make a diagnosis of OCD and ADD, all other psychiatric disorders that might cause OCD or ADD must be ruled out.

The patient satisfies the DSM-IV criteria for panic disorder. The patient has a 3 to 4 year history of panic attacks, as many as three per day and as few as one per month. The patient has fears of leaving her house and avoids school.

The patient's motor restlessness and distractibility stem from anxiety. The patient's obsessive thoughts about health also stem from panic attacks, causing her fear of dying.

Differential Diagnosis

The possible causes of the patient's obsessive thoughts and inattentiveness include:

1. OCD and ADD
2. Schizophrenia
3. Panic disorder
4. Mood disorder
5. Substance abuse
6. Others

The patient has no history of substance abuse, no psychosis that might relate to schizophrenia. Her mood is stabilized with Tegretol. The patient's psychiatric exam is consistent with anxiety disorder, and she satisfies the DSM-IV criteria for panic disorder. Treatment of the panic disorder eventually controls the patient's symptoms.

Appendix N
Case Study of Panic Disorder

A 22-year-old white male presents with the chief complaint of chest pain and shortness of breath twice a month. The patient satisfies the DSM-IV criteria for panic disorder.

History includes six panic attacks during a 2-month period at age 16. During the past month, the patient has had four panic attacks (one per week). The patient has anticipatory anxiety about leaving his house and avoids all social events. The patient has never been treated for a psychiatric disorder. The patient's physical exam and lab work are within normal limits.

The patient has no drug history, including alcohol and amphetamines. The patient is single and a graduate student in physics. His hobbies include snow skiing and weightlifting. The patient has support systems in place, including his parents who assist him with school expenses.

Psychiatric exam reveals a calm 22-year-old male. His manner is friendly. Appearance is neat, healthy, and hygienic. His mood is euthymic. His affect is full range. Motor level is normal. No overt psychosis is present. The patient is alert, oriented to time, place, and person. His recent and remote memory function is normal. Note the patient's psychiatric exam is normal, which is *not* unusual for panic disorder diagnosis.

Family history is positive for panic disorder (maternal aunt).

The patient's life is balanced and it is likely that symptoms stem from biological determinants.

Discussion/Diagnosis

The patient has typical symptoms of panic disorder, no drug abuse, and a positive family history for panic disorder. The patient has the common sequence of symptoms:

1. Panic attacks
2. Anticipatory anxiety
3. Avoidance behavior

The differential diagnosis in this case includes:

1. Drug abuse (with the result that drug withdrawal may cause panic attacks)
2. Thyroid disease, i.e., hypothyroidism
3. A component of another psychiatric disease, as seen when a schizophrenic panics in response to paranoia
4. Severe stress reaction

Treatment

1. Block anxiety attacks
2. Desensitive patient to anticipatory anxiety and avoidance behavior using step-by-step approach for overcoming anxiety
3. Educate the patient about the mechanisms of illness, including the "on-off" switch in the brain stem. Medical therapy is directed to keep the "off" switch on "off," or to prevent the switch from spontaneously going to "on."

Appendix O
Case Study of Alcoholism

A 50-year-old divorced male, who lives alone, presents with "depression." The patient does not meet the DSM-IV criteria for major depression, but has features of depression, including depressed mood, anxiety, and insomnia. The patient has work-related stress, particularly with regard to being overlooked for a promotion at the utility company where he works. The patient works in a middle management position and has a college degree in business. The patient has been socially isolated. His hobbies (tennis) have been abandoned. The patient's health has worsened with weight gain and hypertension. His habits include four or more martinis per night and more drinking on the weekends. The patient has no history of psychiatric or alcohol treatment. The patient's family history is positive for alcoholism (mother and maternal grandfather). He has two children in college.

Neurological exam reveals a nervous white male. Pulse is 100. Blood pressure is 150/100; both readings are increased due to alcohol withdrawal. His gait is slightly unsteady because of the effects of alcohol on the cerebellum. Outstretched hands show a fine tremor. The skin on his chest shows spider nevi. His liver is enlarged. His abdomen is obese.

Psychiatric exam reveals a hyperalert and nervous white male. The patient is slightly disheveled and appears ill (alcohol makes people ill). Mood is depressed. Affect is constricted. No psychosis is present. The patient is hesitant and exhibits poor speech and recent memory. The patient has a difficult time concentrating. The patient denies suicidal thoughts.

The patient's behavioral problems are determined by two determinants—alcoholism and severe psychosocial stress.

Discussion/Diagnosis

The patient has two reinforcing behavioral vectors. The alcohol promotes social isolation and depression. The patient's social isolation promotes increased depression and use of alcohol. Even though the patient denies suicidal thoughts, he is a high risk for suicide if action is not taken to help him.

Neurological and psychiatric exams are consistent with alcoholism. The patient's physical status reflects overuse of alcohol. The patient's laboratory results reflect an alcohol-induced hepatitis.

The differential diagnosis involves an examination of all the motivators that involve alcohol use:

1. Self-medication of mood disorder
2. Abnormal content of life, i.e., PTSD
3. Maladaptive behaviors that cause psychological stress
4. Lack of spirituality

Treatment

The focus of treatment is the patient's alcoholism, which is a medical disorder that is treated nonmedically. The patient is referred to an outpatient alcoholic program, including an Alcoholics Anonymous (AA) 12-Step program. The patient is treated for alcohol withdrawal, which is independent of his alcoholism. The mechanism for withdrawal is different from the mechanism of addiction.

Psychosocial stress, including social isolation, is another focus of therapy. The AA 12-Step program and attendance at AA meetings will help. The patient is referred for psychotherapy to enhance his coping skills and strategies of life. Antidepressants will not be used unless his symptoms persist despite AA meetings, sobriety, and psychotherapy.

After the patient stabilizes his drinking and begins psychotherapy, health maintenance issues are significant. The patient receives instruction with regard to:

1. diet for nutrition and weight loss
2. exercise for cardiovascular effects and general health
3. the importance of regular sleep.

Appendix P
Case Study of Behavior Generated Independent of Personality

A 45-year-old white female presents with chief complaint of "depression." The patient has no history of depression except for the current 1-month-long incident, which is accompanied by low self-esteem, low energy, early morning awakening, and agitation. The patient is so depressed that she has taken medical leave from work. She denies suicidal thoughts and does not have a history of suicidal behavior.

The patient satisfies the DSM-IV criteria for major depression. Her social stressors are low. She has no history of drug abuse or head trauma. Her medical history is negative. She has yearly physical examinations with normal PAP smears. The patient has been married for 20 years and works as an office administrator. She has no history of hypomania. She has a strong spiritual base and volunteers for her church.

Psychiatric exam reveals a slightly disheveled white female who speaks in a nervous manner. Her health and hygiene are good. Her mood is depressed. Her affect is constricted. Motor level is increased, or agitated. No overt psychosis is present. She is alert, oriented to time, place, and person. She exhibits good recent and remote memory function. Neurological exam is normal. Family history is positive for depression; her mother had two bouts of depression during her lifetime.

Discussion

The patient presents with depression. The chief complaint maps into a behavioral cluster for major depression, which defines brain dysfunction. The patient has a balanced life with no excessive stress; she does not abuse drugs. Medical exam, laboratory exams, and neurological exams are normal. The mental status exam is consistent with depression. Family history indicates a genetic vulnerability for depression. There is a high probability that a biological determinant is causing her behavioral problem.

Treatment

The patient is diagnosed with major depression, first episode. Her treatment plan includes:

1. Antidepressant
2. Psychotherapy
   - Educational program (patient and family)
   - Suicide prevention
   - Support

In this case, all psychotherapy is adjunctive to support the medical treatments. If specific maladaptive behavioral problems persist after recovery, the patient will be referred for psychotherapy. The patient is taught the neuropsychiatric model of the brain and how to identify illness behavior versus behavior relating to personality.

The patient's illness behavior is generated independent of personality and content of life. All the behavior within the illness cluster can be identified within the awareness center. Once the patient recovers, relapse prevention will be a goal.

Appendix Q
Case Study of Marital Discord (featuring demonstration of the Open Model)

A married couple presents with the chief complaint of "being separated for 6 months." They have been married for 6 years. The husband is a 45-year-old physician who works as an internist. The wife is a 40-year-old office administrator. Their 2-year-old son lives with the wife.

The husband's chief complaint about his wife is her anger. The wife has a history of cyclical periods of decreased sleep, mood swings, and excessive spending. Evaluation of the wife reveals a bipolar Type II disorder based on a positive family history, early onset of cyclical mood swings, and negative drug use. Physical and neurological exams are negative. The source of the wife's excessive anger is her bipolar disorder.

The wife's chief complaint about her husband is that he is rigid, obsessive about his work, and has difficulty being on time. Evaluation of the husband reveals obsessive-compulsive disorder (OCD) based on positive family history, and the patient satisfies the DSM-IV criteria for OCD. Physical and neurological exams are negative.

The couple is educated about the neuropsychiatric model of the brain. Specifically, the wife is shown how her mood disorder causes emotional overreactivity (anger). The husband is shown how his OCD causes emotional rigidity and obsessiveness. He is shown that he obsesses so much in preparing for social events or air travel that he is late for events or misses plane flights.

Treatment

1. Both husband and wife are treated in an attempt to stop the independent generators of behavior that interfere with their relationship. The wife is treated with Depakole to stabilize her bipolar disorder. The husband is treated with Prozac to stabilize his OCD.

2. Evaluation is performed with regard to the way in which illness behavior disrupts interpersonal relationships. The husband's obsessiveness causes him to be codependent, focusing on his wife's priorities, needs, and desires because she has become distant and less intimate. Also, the husband resents his wife because he makes what he considers to be a significant effort in the relationship (to an obsessive degree), but there are no improvements.

The wife has become less intimate because she has excessive anger. The reinforcing behaviors manifested by her and her husband have caused their marital incompatibility. Despite both parties' desire to make their relationship succeed, they cannot.

3. Both parties are referred for individual therapy—the husband for behavioral treatment targeting OCD and codependence, and the wife for behavioral treatment for anger control. Both parties also are referred for couples therapy to reestablish the relationship, to facilitate communication, understanding, and intimacy.

Discussion

It is important to note that brain disorders are not disorders of will or self-control. This couple cannot "will" their relationship to be normal. This case demonstrates the open model of the brain. The source of interpersonal difficulties is the biology of each individual involved, while the consequences include harm to the personal psychology of both parties and the dynamics of their relationship.

	Biology	*Biology*	
Biological psychiatrist	Bipolar disorder	OCD	Biological psychiatrist
	Psychology	*Psychology*	
Behavioral therapist	Anger, lack of capacity for intimacy	Codependence, resentment of partner	Biological therapist
	Dynamics (behavior between two or more individuals)		
	Marital therapy	Marital discord	

Biological psychiatrists must understand the psychological and dynamic ramifications of OCD and mood disorders, while therapists must understand the biological sources of the behaviors they treat. The multimodality approach (open model) gives the best results, although the complexity of behavior makes problem-solving difficult.

Appendix R
Case Study of Misdiagnosed Dementia and Depression

A 75-year-old man is asked to be seen for severe dementia and depression. The patient had a stroke at age 73 involving his right brain, which resulted in left-sided weakness. The patient has a history of small transient strokes. Since his stroke the patient has a history of withdrawal, tearfulness, and being noncommunicative. The patient has no history of psychiatric disorders and has been in good health up until his stroke. Medical evaluation is negative except for stroke. The patient's family history is negative for psychiatric conditions, including depression. Drug use, including over-the-counter and illicit types, is negative. The patient takes one aspirin each day.

Psychiatric exam reveals a white male sitting in a wheelchair. The patient spontaneously moves his right hand but must exert great effort to move his left hand. The patient's speech is inarticulate, i.e., it requires great effort to articulate words. The patient spontaneously cries and grimaces. In spite of the patient's tearfulness, however, he denies being depressed. The patient states that his emotional outbursts are not under his control and his tearfulness occurs in spite of feeling normal.

Psychiatric exam reveals a white male who spontaneously cries. The patient's appearance is disheveled. Manner is abrupt with surges of tearfulness or grimacing. His speech is abrupt and hard to understand. Mood is euthymic. Affect is highly restricted. Motor level is less on the weak left side. No psychosis is present. The patient is oriented to time, place, and person. Mini mental status exam is 30 out of 30.

Discussion and Treatment

The patient's diagnosis is not dementia because of the patient's score (30 out of 30) on the mini mental status exam. The patient is not depressed nor does he satisfy the DSM-IV criteria for major depression. The patient's new diagnosis is pseudobulbar palsy, which is a disconnection syndrome.

The patient's strokes disconnected his emotional state from the facial expressions that appropriately represent emotional states. Medications may be helpful.

Appendix S
Common Psychiatric Medications*
(Brand names listed on left, generic
names listed on right)

Selective serotonergic reuptake inhibitors (antidepressants)

Prozac	fluoxetine
Zoloft	sertraline
Luvox	fluoxamine
Paxil	paroxetine

Mood stabilizers

Eskalith	lithium carbonate

Monoaminoxidase inhibitors (MAOIs/antidepressants)

Nardil	phenelzine
Parnate	tranylcypromine

Anticonvulsants/mood stabilizers

Depakote	valproic acid
Tegretol	carbamazepine

Tricyclic antidepressants

Tofranil	imipramine
Anafranil	clomipramine

Selective norepinephrine uptake blockers/antidepressants

Wellbutrin	bupropion

Selective norephinephrine and serotonin uptake blockers/antidepressants

Effexor	venlafaxine

Antipsychotics

Risperdal	risperidone
Zypexa	olansepine

Benzodiazepines/antianxiety medications

Valium	diazepam
Ativan	lorazepam
Librium	chlordiazepoxide
Xanax	alprazolam
Klonopin	clonazepam

*Medications can be classified according to (a) the impact they have on **behavior** (i.e., mood stabilizers or antidepressants), (b) their **structure** (i.e., tricyclic antidepressants, where "tricyclic" means that three cyclical rings comprise the basic structure of the drug), and (3) the **pharmalogical actions** of the drug (i.e., selective serotonin reuptake inhibitors, where "selective" means that the drug selects only serotonin to inhibit reuptake).

Appendix T
Comprehensive treatment involving the five variables that affect mood

The following is an example of the way in which different forms of treatment are used together in treating a menopausal, bipolar patient with a history of diabetes. Note that treatment requires a team of professionals comprised (in this example) of a biological psychiatrist, psychologist, dietitian, internist, and physical therapist.

Symptom	Treatment
Cycling of illness	Lithium carbonate pulls the cycles apart and decreases the intensity of symptoms and chances of relapse
Seasonal affect	During winter depressions bright light therapy is used in the early morning
Hormonal fluctuation	Replacement hormones prescribed by a gynecologist would be used because of meno-pausal symptoms
Stress	Health maintenance and psychotherapy monitored by a psychologist
Other illnesses (diabetes)	An internist would treat dia-betes with diet (monitored by a dietitian), insulin and a course of exercise (moni-tored by a physical therapist)

Glossary

Aberration: A small amount of abnormal behavior that does not significantly affect normal brain function.

Abuse: Any physical or psychological stress that is unwanted.

Acute confusion state: Sudden, diffuse metabolic dysfunction that presents primarily with confusion and memory loss.

Addiction: A medical disorder of the brain caused by activation of an inherently vulnerable generator of behavior that has the capacity to create behavior independent of personality behavior. As a result of repeated use of a substance not normally needed for sustenance, the vulnerable generator of behavior creates a craving for the same substance. Use of the substance and/or associated behaviors interferes with normal functioning.

Affective disorder: Characterized by disturbance in affect or the way individuals cyclically experience mood (i.e., depression, manic disorder).

Alzheimer's disease: A primary type of dementia that causes progressive degeneration of memory and other behaviors, usually in elderly individuals.

Antisocial personality disorder (sociopathy): Has a strong genetic determinant, is evident on a constant basis and has no known treatment; characterized by lack of conscience, and inability to maintain social norms related to humanistic values.

Anxiety disorder: Marked by physical and psychological symptoms that occur during a definite period of time—rapid pulse, pounding heart, chest pain, sweating, nausea, diarrhea, and feelings of panic (i.e., phobia's, anxiety state, posttraumatic stress disorder).

Aphophanous phenomena: Another term for "belief disturbance."

Attention deficit disorder (ADD): Characterized by distractibility, inattentiveness, poor planning capacity, and impaired ability to execute and follow through on tasks.

Awareness: Sustained reflective thought that is produced in response to information received in the brain's awareness center, the part of the brain that creates a sense of existence.

Awareness array: The series of types of awareness that correspond to subjective assignments—sensory, instinctive, working memory, spiritual, and others. The awareness array is much like a blackboard, and the disconnection of various inputs to awareness is like erasing the board. Meditation (which is induced by

285

exercising executive function to focus on spiritual awareness) allows the board to be cleaned. When the nervous system awareness center is bombarded with input, meditation eliminates the input and facilitates an inner calm.

Awareness, external: Awareness of input or stimuli that is generated outside the brain.

Awareness, internal: Awareness of input or stimuli generated within the brain.

Behavior: Anything that reflects brain activity.

Behavior, aberrant: Activity produced when an independent generator produces non-disruptive behavior, i.e., an aberration.

Behavior, abnormal: Results when brain failure occurs, which affects normal brain functioning.

Behavior, addictive: Occurs when part of the brain is challenged by a particular substance and an unnatural independent generator of behavior emerges.

Behavior, maladaptive (neurosis): Reflects personality behavior, not illness behavior, that is counter-productive to patient's goals.

Behavior, metabolic: Reflects the rate of brain cell metabolism.

Behavior, neuroendocrine: Reflects the brain's hypothalmic pituitary activity.

Behavior, normal: Occurs when all behavioral areas function well.

Behavior, overt: Brain activity that can be observed without special equipment; the primary form of functional behavior.

Behavioral therapy: Therapy that emphasizes "unlearning" of poor behavioral habits through setting achievable goals and working toward them gradually.

Belief disturbance: One of the four traditional psychoses, as seen with delusions.

Body dysmorphic disorder (BDD): Involves the way individuals perceive themselves, causing obsessive thoughts about suspected defects in appearance.

Biological approach: Method of psychiatric assessment and treatment based on the premise that all behavior is biologically based.

Biological health field: All the professions that are involved with assessment and treatment of the three primary categories of behavioral determinants. These include medical doctors and biological psychiatrists (biological determinants), psychologists and therapists (psychosocial determinants), and members of the clergy (spiritual determinants).

Borderline personality disorder (BPD): Marked by a pattern of instability in interpersonal relationships and self-image, as well as extreme impulsivity.

Brain failure (psychosis): Behavior that represents brain dysfunction that is physiologically based and treatable with medical therapy.

Brain model: A diagrammatic way of viewing the brain and behavior, based on scientific data, observed data and intuitive thought.

Breathing-related sleep disorder: Disrupts sleep and causes daytime sleepiness (obstructive sleep apnea is the most common type).

Bright light therapy: Therapy that utilizes exposure to bright light and is most effective in treating seasonal affective disorder and delayed sleep phase syndrome.

Chief complaint: A patient's problem, stated: in his or her own words.

Circadian rhythm: The sleep-wake cycle.

Circadian rhythm disorder: A recurrent pattern of sleep disruption that results from a mismatch between circadian sleep-wake system and demands regarding timing and duration of sleep.

Circumstantial thoughts: Characterized by responses (during the Mental Status Exam) given by the patient that include excessive wording or irrelevant information.

Codependence: Behavior characterized by: (a) focus on another individual's priorities, (b) lack of healthy personal boundaries, and (c) decreased capacity to communicate needs.

Cognitive functioning: Determined by asking specific questions on the standardized Mini-Mental Status Exam (part of the MSE).

Cognitive therapy: Therapy that emphasizes modification of thought processes in order to change mood or other behaviors.

Conversion disorder (also known as "Temporary Disconnection Syndrome or TDS): An anxiety disorder that affects neurological capacities, presumably by disconnection from awareness and executive capacity.

Coping skills: Different psychological mechanisms that relate to the ability to deal with stress.

Core beliefs: Long-standing beliefs (held since childhood) that have become structurally integrated into the personality.

Counseling: An educational process to provide information to patients and address multiple issues; designed to help patients develop treatment strategies and informed expectations about treatment.

Culpable: Deserving blame, blameworthy.

Cyclical variable: Behavioral determinant that tends to cycle or follow a predictable pattern.

Delirium: Diffuse metabolic dysfunction that presents primarily with agitation and hallucinations.

Delirium/Encephalopathy: An acute diffuse process that involves inattention, rambling speech and other brain problems.

Delusion: A fixed false belief.

Dementia: Characterized by loss of cognitive function, usually starting with memory disturbance and progressing to psychosis (i.e., Alzheimer's disease).

Depression: Mood disorder marked by low energy, slowed thinking, and low self-esteem (i.e., low brain activation).

Derailment: Characterized by rapidly jumping from one idea to the next, reflected during the Mental Status Exam.

Deviant belief behavior: Takes the form of beliefs that are not false but deviate from socially acceptable belief.

Diagnosis: Phases of analysis and testing of symptoms, based on the medical model, that lead to identification and treatment of illness.

Diagnosis, differential: Multiple diagnostic possibilities.

Diagnosis, provisional: A tentative diagnosis.

Disorder of experience (also known as "first rank symptom"): One of the four traditional psychoses, as seen when an individual feels as though his or her body is being controlled by outside forces.

Double-blind placebo: A controlled scientific study where illness evaluators and patients are "blind" to the active ingredient in a medication, as being a placebo ("sugar pill") or "active" medication.

Dysphoria: An abnormal ill feeling.

Eating disorder: Characterized by eating behavioral disturbances and usually presents in one of three forms:
- **Bulimia nervosa**: Involves binge eating with compensatory behavior (i.e., self-induced vomiting, use of laxatives).
- **Anorexia nervosa** is a severe internal perceptual disorder, resulting in dysphoria with loss of appetite.
- **Obesity**: Involves excessive eating.

Electroconvulsive therapy: Therapy that utilizes electrical stimulation (in conjunction with anesthesia and relaxation therapy) in treating psychosis.

Electroencephalogram: The primary method of measuring the brain's electrical activity.

Encephalopathy: Diffuse metabolic dysfunction that presents primarily with decreased alertness.

Existence: The interaction of mass, energy, and time particles.

Experience of influencing: The experience of feeling that the body is controlled by external forces (i.e., as a robot).

50 (Fifty)-Second Hour: A method of diagnosis that can be made in 50 seconds in the family practice or internal medicine setting.

Fixed false belief behavior: Takes the form of delusions, which indicate brain failure.

Formal thought disorder: One of the four traditional psychoses, reflected in higher language disorders.

General anxiety disorder (GAD): An anxiety disorder that is marked by continuous apprehensive expectation.

Generator of behavior: Any one of a group of behavioral elements that comprises the personality matrix, i.e., groups of neurons that have a common function.

Gestalt experience: A "total" experience; more than just the summation of the individual parts of experience.

Greed: The tendency to hoard material good, which is motivated by instinct as well as social values. Greed may promote antisocial behavior.

Helplessness: The perception that there is no ability to think or perform a task.

Hopelessness: The perception that there is no hope for the future.

Hypochondriasis: A preoccupation with fears of having a serious disease.

Illness: A disorder related to brain dysfunction that is chronic, occurs apart from life circumstances or personality, and disrupts functioning.

Illness behavior: Generated by an inherent vulnerability in the brain, this activity creates one or more independent generators of behavior that interfere with normal brain function.

Independent generator of behavior: Any one or more of the behavioral generators that comprise personality, which pulls away from the personality matrix, functions independent of normal brain capacity, and causes brain dysfunction.

Insertion: The experience that one's thoughts are not one's own (i.e., someone else's thoughts are being inserted into one's mind).

Instinct: Preprogrammed behavior.

Interacting syndromes: Occur when one condition worsens another condition by creating physiological stress, or "overlapping symptoms."

Integrated approach (to psychiatry): Consideration of all major determinants of behavior.

Internist: Specialist in the field of internal medicine, a division of medicine that focuses on *medical*, not surgical, treatment of medical disorders.

Interpersonal therapy: Therapy that emphasizes social relationship and communication skills by focusing on dynamic behavior between two or more individuals.

Issue: Term used by psychologists or therapists to refer to psychological matters related to either current or past content-of-life problems.

Kindling: The behavioral affect that occurs when brain cells that cause abnormal function at a quickened pace (as *kindling* wood is used to rapidly start a fire), which can lead to progression of illness or other diseases.

Major brain disorder: Classification of abnormality that is most common and has the potential to cause severe symptoms or suicide.

Maladaptive belief behavior: Involves beliefs that are not known to be false but are intensely defended and often are accompanied by maladaptive behavioral response.

Malingering: Reporting (by the patient) of false information about symptoms for the purpose of secondary gain.

Mania: Mood disorder marked by high energy, sharpened thinking, and high self-esteem (i.e., enhanced brain activation)

Medical incompetence: The condition that exists when neurological dysfunction is present, which can interfere with the normal processes that are involved with medical decision-making.

Medical model: The scientific and rational approach to understanding and defining illness as well as treatment of illness.

Meditation: The exercise of executive function that provides a sustained focus on spiritual awareness. It allows disconnection from other inputs to awareness.

Mental Status Examination (MSE): A test designed to assess current behavior based on systematic observation of overt behavior.

Mixed mood state: Characterized by symptoms of both depression and mania.

Model: A simple representation of the way in which variables in a system interact.

Mood: The underlying and dominant psychological state that exists independent of reactivity.

Narcolepsy: Involves the onset of sleep during awake periods.

Nervous breakdown (a term commonly used by patients but not yet scientifically defined): Denotes the point at which a patient becomes so agitated that he or she is no longer able to cope with his or her illness.

Neuron: The brain's fundamental structural element, comprised of a soma (cell body), a series of dendrites, an axon and an area of pre- and postsynaptic terminals.

Neuropsychiatric brain model (Williams Brain Model): A model of the brain that explains illness behavior, awareness, and other sources of behavior.

Neuropsychiatry: Science of the brain and behavior.

Neurosis: Maladaptive behavior that occurs simultaneously with normal brain function.

Neurotransmitter: A modified amino acid or other substance that allows for transmission of information between neurons by direct diffusion and interaction.

Nightmare disorder: Consists of repeated frightening dreams that may lead to awakenings.

Observed behavior: Activity noted (during the Mental Status Exam) by observation of appearance, mood/affect/anxiety level and motor level.

Obsessive compulsive disorder (OCD): Involves excessive instinctual behavior (i.e., excessive handwashing or hair-pulling, checking) that results in obsessive thoughts, compulsions.

Open model: The overarching framework used to define and treat illness, which includes other models, such as:
- the medical model and applications to biological psychiatry
- psychological models that have varying scientific bases
- the spiritual model, which has no scientific basis

Overlapping syndromes: Created when two or more independent generators occur simultaneously.

Pain disorder: Results from normal integration of pain and causes disruption of behavioral functioning.

Panic disorder: An anxiety disorder caused by a defect in the brain stem mechanism that controls response to perceived danger and causes random panic attacks.

Perceptual disturbance: One of the four traditional psychoses, as seen with hallucinations.

Personality: Comprised of a combination of all individual generators of behavior that overlap and create a composite of behavior.

Personality disorders: Inflexible and maladaptive patterns of perception, relative to the environment and the self, that cause significant functional impairment.

Pervasive developmental disorders: Characterized by onset of severe and progressive impairment during childhood, in many areas of development. These include:

- **Autistic disorder**: Early onset brain dysfunction that affects social interaction, language, and play
- **Rett's disorder**: Development of multiple deficits after a period of normal function following birth, found only in females
- **Childhood disintegrative disorder (CDD)**: Marked by regression in multiple areas of function, following at least 2 years of apparently normal development, associated with severe mental retardation and high incident of seizure disorder
- **Asperger's disorder**: Characterized by severe, sustained impairment of social interaction and development of restricted patterns of behavior, interests, and activities

Positron Emission Tomography (PET): Diagnostic brain scan that measures metabolic activity of neurons.

Posttraumatic stress disorder (PTSD): An anxiety disorder marked by dysfunctional memory caused by severe stress-induced anxiety.

Primary hypersomnia: Involves prolonged sleep episodes.

Primary insomnia: Caused by a weak sleep generator.

Primary sleep disorder: Related to an inherent problem in the sleep-regulating system and can be divided into two categories:

- **Dyssomnias**: Caused by a disturbance in the amount, quality or timing sleep.
- **Parasomnias**: Characterized by abnormal behavior or psychological events during sleep.

Psychoanalysis: Therapy that is based on dealing with unconscious conflicts that impair normal brain function.

Psychosis: Any overt behavior that clearly represents brain dysfunction and impedes normal human functioning with regard to self and/or interpersonal, social, or work relationships and activities.

Psychosocial disorder: Brain dysfunction characterized by stress as the primary determinant.

Psychosomatic brain dysfunction: Brain disorder that occurs due to various forms of stress, not illness; may be generated by exceptional external stressors (i.e., drugs) that cause normal generators of behavior to malfunction.

Psychosomatic disorder: Disorder of the body (not the brain) characterized by stress as the primary determinant of body dysfunction.

Psychotherapy: Therapy in which the mind itself is the major determinant of behavioral change.

Queried behavior: Behavior noted during the Mental Status Exam by asking general questions that might reveal one of the four traditional psychoses.

Sleep disorder: Anything that disturbs sleep and prevents normal functioning.

Schizophrenia, disorganized type: Characterized by catatonic behavior.

Schizophrenia, paranoid type: Characterized by delusions, hallucinations, and disorganized speech.

Schizophrenic disorder: Caused by a combination of temporal lobe overactivity (causing delusions or hallucinations) and/or frontal lobe underactivity (causing social isolation or emotional blunting).

Seasonal affective disorder (SAD): A mood disorder that occurs in response to varying lengths of day, i.e., winter depression.

Self-monitoring methods: Techniques by which patients can recognize their illness behavior, utilizing internal awareness of illness behavior and external awareness of illness consequences. By helping patients discriminate between normal personality behavior and illness behavior, self-monitoring techniques are specifically designed to enhance the capacity to *control* illness.

Sleep terror disorder: Comprised of repeated episodes of sleep terrors during which there is autonomic arousal and intense fear, accompanied by screaming, crying, or incoherent vocalization.

Sleep walking disorder: Consists of repeated episodes of complex motor behavior (i.e., walking) during sleep.

Signs and symptoms: Behavioral characteristics that manifest the presence of brain failure; signs are elements that can be observed by the physician, while symptoms are subjective complaints made by the patient.

Social phobia: Involves the social instinct of being watched and judged by others, causing severe anxiety and fear.

Somatization disorder: Involves the instinct to integrate and feel pain, causing an individual to experience pain in a diffuse manner.

Specific lobe dysfunction: Occurs when there is failure of a well defined area, or lobe, of the brain that controls a particular function.

Spirituality: The personal quest for inner peace, as well as relation-ships of depth and relevancy with other individuals.

Strategies of life: All options and combinations of options that may lead to different outcomes of life.

Stress model: Framework that connects content of life and brain physiology by increasing and decreasing the threshold for illness symptoms.

Structural disorders: Caused by direct physical contact (i.e., stroke or trauma) or direct toxic contact (i.e., alcohol or dry addiction).

Tangential thoughts: Characterized by responses (during the Mental Status Exam) where the patient talks around the main point and never arrives at the answer.

Thought broadcasting: The experience that thoughts are being "broadcast" from the head (i.e., radio waves).

Traditional psychosis: Behavior that is observably abnormal in one of four areas—thought disorder, belief disorder, perceptual disorder, or disorder of experience.

Vegetative state: A condition that exists when a patient has no cortical awareness and exists on hypothalamic and brain stem function only. Often produced by head trauma and strokes.

Will: The use of executive function in the frontal lobes to control behavior.

Williams Brain Model (Neuropsychiatric brain model): A schematic representation of illness.

Williams 5-Part Psychiatric Plan: Part of the Williams 10-Step Evaluation Process; the 5-Part Plan is used to effect treatment.

Williams 5-Step Approach to Treatment: The 5-step approach to treatment, based on the medical model.

Williams 10-Step Evaluation Process: A method of diagnosing organ system failure, based on the open model.

Working memory: This type of memory allows choices: and the weighted subjective assignments for those choices. An individual can experience and "slide" executive function from one choice to the other; the strongest subjective sense attracts the individual to a particular choice. There can be a decision to accept the choice, reevaluate, gather more information for working memory, or stop the process of making a choice. The interaction of working memory and awareness facilitate recognition of the decision-making process. Will allow the intact process of executive decision-making to function and to be a focus of behavior.

Index

About the Author

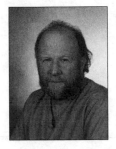

Dr. Robert A. Williams was born October 26, 1942 in San Francisco, California, and grew up in Piedmont, California. He graduated from California High School in Whittier, California in 1960. Dr. Williams graduated from the University of California-Berkeley in 1964 with a degree in Zoology and was a member of the Phi Kappa Tau fraternity. In 1967, Dr. Williams graduated from San Jose State University with a Masters Degree in Physical Science. While in college, he completed an ROTC program and was commissioned as a 2nd Lieutenant in the U.S. Army in 1967. Dr. Williams served 2 years in the army from 1967 to 1969 as a missile scientist at the White Sands Missile Range in New Mexico. He received his Medical Doctorate from the University of New Mexico in Albuquerque in 1974.

Dr. Williams served his internship in Neurology at the University of New Mexico. His computer background includes his Masters Thesis, "Automatiion and Its Software Applications to System Sensitivities," submitted at New Mexico State University-Las Cruces in 1969, and a medical school course, "Computers in Clinical Medicine," in 1972 at the Division of Research and Technology (DCRT) of the National Institute of Health in Bethesda, Maryland.

Dr. Williams spent 3 years in emergency medicine, including 1 year in Tabuk, Saudi Arabia. He completed his psychiatric residency in 1982 and his neurology residency in 1983 at the Chicago Medical School. Dr. Williams participated in 1 year of clinical research involving electroconvulsive therapy (ECT) and was coauthor of two publications on ECT.

Dr. Williams was clinical director of the Affective Disorders Clinic at Maricopa Medical Center in Phoenix, Arizona, from 1983 to 1987. From 1987 to the present, Dr. Williams has been the director of the Biological Psychiatry Institute in Phoenix. He was medical director of the geropsychiatric inpatient unit at Phoenix Baptist Hospital from 1992 until the unit was closed in 1995. He currently provides an introductory course, "Introduction to Biological Psychiatry," to the family practice residents at Phoenix Baptist Hospital.

Dr. Williams is a Unitarian Universalist with hobbies that include art and photography. He spends his free time hiking and vacationing at his mountain residence in Pinos Altos, New Mexico.